Living Thin
In A
Fast Food World

*How To Lose Weight
& Stay That Way*

**The Use-Anywhere Guide To
Modern Diet,
Nutrition and Exercise**

Jill-Anne Bennett, MD.

NMD Books
Simi Valley, CA

Visit our Web site at http://www.NMDbooks.com.

Library of Congress Cataloging-in-Publication Data
Living Thin In A Fast Food World by Jill-Anne Bennett
Includes bibliographical references and index.

ISBN: 978-0-9706773-7-2 (Softcover)

First Edition August 2010

Table of Contents

APPENDIX

Why I Wrote This Book – And Why You Need It

Nobody likes being overweight, except maybe Sumo wrestlers, and I suspect even they aren't too happy about it. So why is it that after all these years, all the diet books, the endless weight-loss programs, and all the proven methods and research about losing weight do we continue to go down the same path of least resistance, overeat, procrastinate, then end up buying yet another diet book?

I asked myself that question over and over, trying to come up with an answer that made sense, and then, trying to come up with a way to offer a solution to that dilemma that was both sensible and simple, yet unique.

But, fact is, there is nothing really new under the sun about losing weight. As much as we might like to believe, no magic bullet seems to be emerging from the scientific community, although the hucksters and marketers and infomercials would have us believe otherwise.

'Calories in and calories out' is the same principle now as it always has been. The way to lose weight is to consistently burn more calories than you consume. Nothing new about that.

What is new and unique is our modern diet. Fast food restaurants, coupled with the processed foods industry have turned us into a race of unhealthy, overweight slugs.

It seems there is little that can be done to stop the tide.

But, there is a solution rather than giving up the fight for fitness.

That solution starts with this book.

The knowledge you will gain from this guide may not be groundbreaking science, or offer a quick easy fix to a problem that has been growing for decades.

But it *is* knowledge you can use to take small steps toward making big changes.

In writing this book, my goal was to take popular misconceptions about weight-loss and expose them as false; to review common mistakes made by many and turn them toward more healthy eating behaviors; and to create a guide that can be taken anywhere and used on the spot to make more healthful choices.

Pretty cool, huh?

I also wanted to present the information in a fun, "easy to digest" (pun intended) format, using humor and thought-provoking wit all along the way. After all, it's about the journey not just the destination, right?

So we are going to enjoy the ride, whether you like it or not.

At best, the book you now hold in your hands just may be the most important and life-changing book you will ever own. At worst, it may simply remind you that losing weight is not easy, you'd rather couch it with a bag of chips and some ice cream, and may end up in the bargain bin of your local Thrift Store.

(Where it could then lead a second life as the catalyst for making some budding fitness guru the next Richard Simmons, so be careful where you leave this book lying around)

Use this book as a reminder, a guide to living and a working tool to accomplish the most basic goal we have as human beings: to maximize our health and be comfortable and healthy in our bodies.

What's So Great About Overweight?

There was a time in history when overweight was fashionable, back when the Romans liked their partners plump and painters immortalized them in lusty frescoes of fruit, frolic and just plain nastiness.

Back and forth over the ages, it seemed like 'thin was in,' and even recently we've been conditioned to believe that the accepted norm for body image are heroin tainted waifs gazing out at us with ghoulish hollowed-out eyes from the pages of fashion magazines and Times Square billboards.

Well, guess what? Popular fashion and good health make strange bedfellows.

Then there are the overweight stars who celebrate their weight problems by endorsing lines of clothing that cater to similarly-proportioned people, thus perpetuating further another negative body image crisis.

What is truly healthy is not what is being told to you by the media or the fashion industry that is healthy, but by the standards established by the National Institute of Health, and that standard is established (more or less accurately) by the Body Mass Index, or BMI for short.

Our Fast Food Nation – The Grim Statistics

If you already didn't know it, America is overweight, big time. According to the Center for Disease Control and Prevention, about 1/3 of all adults are obese, and slightly over 60% are overweight. These figures showed a sizeable spike in the mid 1980's, when fast food chains began their meteoric growth rates, fueled by corporate dollars and an increasingly mobile and time-pressed society.

Americans have become 'obesogenic,' characterized by environments that promote increased food intake, nonhealthful foods, and physical inactivity.

The increase of junk food has also been accompanied by the fall of the independent farm, forced out of business and replaced by corporate farming conglomerates. The move away from fresh, organic foods and their replacements of pesticide-heavy crops and anti-biotic injected, horribly mistreated livestock has put the nail in our collective coffin.

The rise of processed foods in favor of sugar and flour based empty calories in more and more of our products has not helped the situation.

Couple this with an anxiety driven, time constrained stressed out population now being pressured on all sides by economic and emotional turmoil and it's clear why the common cause of death in this country is heart disease, diabetes and stress. It's also why depression and anxiety are increasing in ever-larger numbers.

There is an answer and it starts with you.

We all make choices in what we eat and how we exercise, and ultimately, how we deal with the world around us.

Rest, Exercise, Diet: The RED Triumvirate

Before we start getting into the nitty-gritty of how all this works, I think it's important to stress the importance of letting you know that it's not just diet and exercise alone that will make you a happier, healthier you.

Much like substance abuse is treated with a combination of modalities to be successful, so we need to treat our own approach to life on multiple fronts. We need to make sure we are doing everything in our lives with moderation and balance.

It is the combination of Mind, Body and Spirit that makes for a more successful and rewarding life, so let's start now to strive for that balance.

I like to use an acronym for RED, because it's easy to remember. In this instance, RED stands for:

R- Rest
E – Exercise
D - Diet

If you will strive to keep a balance of getting the proper rest, regular exercise and maintaining a sensible diet, everything else in your life will fall into place.

Everything is related: You will find if you have trouble with depression, substance abuse, anxiety or other physical and mental difficulties that by maintaining the right RED balance, many if not all of the symptoms of these disorders can be diminished if not completely reversed.

Forget Fear: A Holistic Approach to Health and Well-Being

Fear can be a great motivating factor for losing weight, but for keeping it off, not always. It can work for some, but denial of one's cravings out of fear of a negative result is less desirable than a more holistic and healthy approach to weight control.

As I have mentioned above, the RED approach is a more positive way of approaching weight loss and keeping it off. Visualizing positive outcomes, such as imagining yourself at your ideal weight, feeling healthy, being active, doing things and feeling better about doing them is the better way.

The Ugly Secret About Weight Loss Books – Including This One

Diet and weight control books all harbor one ugly truth: that most people who buy them don't put the information they contain to any real practical use – they put off the work and put the book on a shelf and in the end nothing gets accomplished.

We are going to make a pact, you and I, that you will take small steps toward implementing the techniques in this book in your life, and give it your best effort.

Fact is, the reason why diet books keep coming out is that people are seeking a magic solution to an age-old problem. Bu the books all say the same thing, when it gets right down to it. With very few exceptions, you can lose weight effectively using the techniques in most diet books, at least those that are written by dieticians and physicians and are not proposing a radical and untested and often unhealthy program.

But the reason they keep on coming is that people aren't getting the results they want because they aren't doing the work. Everybody wants the gold but nobody wants to dig!

Results Not Typical:
Facing Hard Truths About Weight Loss An Overview of Commercial Weight Loss Programs - Jenny Craig/Weight Watchers/Nutri-System - What Marie Osmond and Valerie Bertinelli Won't Tell You

Many of the commercial weight loss programs out there basically work on the principle of caloric restriction. No matter how much they package it with fancy commercials and mouth watering photos of delicious looking (but ultimately bland tasting) foods, it all gets down to calories in, calories out.

Most people do not stay on these programs for any real length of time, and do not alter their eating habits and lifestyle to continue the right caloric and metabolic balance. Old habits die hard, and bad food habits are very difficult to overcome.

There is nothing about Jenny Craig, Nutri-System, or any of the weight loss programs being touted by famous actresses that offer any real advantage over the techniques you will find in this book.

What Marie Osmond and Valerie Bertinelli won't tell you is that chances are, after you lose the weight (IF you lose the weight,) you are going to gain it back, which is why every weight loss book and TV commercial you see shows before-and-after photos that in very small print says "results not typical." People KNOW the results shown in the photos are highly unlikely to be achieved, yet the power of belief is a strong motivator.

Unfortunately, the motivation is used to spend money on programs that most likely will not work, and not used to lose the weight itself – and keep it off.

Weight Loss Myths –
How to Create Your Own Success Story

A lot of myths revolve around diets. Some call for carbohydrate restriction, saying they are dangerous and turn to fat. Some myths tell you can never eat the foods you enjoy. Others claim that you have to go to the gym every day.

Other myths revolve around the "ideal weight" principle. What is your ideal weight? It may not be what the experts say.

Information about weight loss can be contradictory and confusing. Even worse, though, are the numerous widely believed weight loss myths. These are a formidable obstacle for people trying to lose weight in a permanent, healthy manner. Here are a few of the more common weight loss myths.

Fad Diets Work

There is no good fad diet. While they often cause weight loss because you're eating less, the weight comes back as soon as the diet is stopped, often with additional weight. In addition, fad diets are all unhealthy.

Cutting Carbs Works

Low-carb, high-protein diets are fad diets, though they've remained popular for many years now. A healthy diet is well balanced, meaning it's inclusive of all the food groups, and is not too disproportionately heavy on one or two groups.

Cut Out Starch

Starches have a bad reputation among dieters, but they're an important low-fat source of complex carbohydrates, a key provider of energy.

Some Foods Burn Fat

Some of the more widely circulated diet myths these days, particularly as part of fad diets, are that certain foods like grapefruit, lemon, celery, cinnamon, chili peppers, and cabbage burn fat. While some (like chili peppers or caffeine) can create a slight, short-lived acceleration of metabolism, no food actually burns fat.

Herbal Weight Loss Products Help

Supplements touting themselves as natural or herbal weight loss products are big business. There is no good evidence that these products have any benefit to dieters, and, more importantly, there are serious, legitimate concerns about their safety.

Creating a success story for yourself means getting down to and maintaining your ideal weight by a sensible exercise and food-planning schedule that's easy to do each day.

You can even take one day a week and eat the foods you crave, if you do it in moderation.

Changing Lifestyle
Doesn't Mean Changing Life

Everybody says "it's a lifestyle change." In some ways it is, particularly if you do not exercise regularly and you are in the habit of eating junk constantly through the day and night. But I maintain that major changes are not needed as much as you might expect or fear.

Weight loss and weight control can be achieved through 30-60 minutes of exercise daily and careful planning of the foods you eat. If you consistently follow the plan each day, even if you are eating out at fast food restaurants, that you'll have to make very changes in your "lifestyle."

Of course, if a major lifestyle is what you'd really like, by all means go for it.

Why Diets Don't Work – and Why Yours Will

When you are losing the weight, sometimes "dieting" is necessary, but once you achieve your ideal weight, this is where the "dieting" element must end and the foods that you used to eat need to be replaced by healthier choices you like, and the foods you crave must be taken in moderation. The key to weight control is to not cut out the foods you crave. This is why a large number of diets don't work. Eventually your cravings for the foods you love overcome your willpower – and we all know willpower doesn't work.

Far From The Maddening Scale – The Numbers Game

The bathroom scale and BMI do not tell the whole story. Every person has a unique and ideal weight that suits their particular body and metabolism. Finding this balance is the key to feeling healthy and maintaining the median weight that's right for you.

Let's use an example. Phil is 50 years old and is 6"1. His BMI is 185lbs, but he has a very difficult time not only getting down to this weight, but also maintaining it.

He has found that his particular body seems to settle in at 200-205lbs, when he is eating right and staying fit. This weight is comfortable for him. His blood sugar levels are normal and his cholesterol numbers are within normal range, and his blood pressure is also within normal range, so maintaining a median weight of 200lbs is right for him.

To be successful at staying thin in a fast food world, you need to find a comfortable median weight average for your body, based on your BMI, your own unique health factors.

Daily and Hourly Weight Fluctuation

How to Understand Daily Weight Fluctuations

I want to do this! What's This?

Many people who are trying to lose weight become needlessly obsessed with daily weight fluctuations. Here's why they occur and why you shouldn't be concerned.

Instructions

Step 1

You've been following your healthy eating plan to the letter and exercising religiously. To your surprise, you step on the scale and are shocked to find you've gained three pounds since yesterday. What's going on? Weight fluctuations are one of the most frustrating aspects of dieting. Just when you're prepared to see the number on the scale drop, it not only doesn't, but also surprises you by adding a few pounds. During these times, it can be reassuring to know that daily weight fluctuations are normal.

Step 2

What causes daily weight fluctuations? Weight fluctuations can be caused by a variety of factors ranging from water retention related to excess salt intake, hormonal changes, constipation, or eating a large meal. Keep in mind that it requires intake of 3,500 calories to gain a pound of body fat and it's unlikely you'll consume that amount in a single day. This is why many dieticians advice patients not to weigh too frequently because the daily weight fluctuations can be discouraging if you take them too seriously.

Step 3

Body weight can vary by as much as five pounds from day to day based on fluid and salt intake and the amount of food still being processed by the digestive system. If you happened to go to a buffet the night before, your weight will probably be up the next morning, particularly if you ate foods high in sodium and haven't had a recent bowel movement. Even if you overindulged a bit, it's unlikely you'll experience a significant increase in true body weight overnight. Real weight gain is a more gradual process.

Step 4

The best way to avoid the stress of daily weight fluctuations is to weigh yourself on a weekly basis. Weigh without clothes or shoes to eliminate the clothing weight which can add up to two pounds. Weigh first thing in the morning after emptying your bladder and bowels to avoid a falsely elevated weight due to food and liquid intake. If you find a weekly weight is elevated, drink lots of water, reduce your salt intake, and reweigh yourself for the next two mornings. If the following two readings are elevated, reassess your eating and exercise habits to make sure you're not taking in too many calories.

Step 5

Be aware of how your clothes are fitting. This can be a more reliable indicator of true weight gain. If you have a scale that measures body fat percentage, look for fluctuations in this value rather than looking at your overall weight, especially if you're doing resistance exercise which can increase lean body mass. Most of all don't let yourself be alarmed by daily weight fluctuations. They're a normal part of living.

Digital VS Analog Scales in Accuracy

At some point you may wonder if there is a difference in accuracy among scales – and the will inevitably lead to an analog vs digital scale debate. Many gyms have analog scales, and your bathroom scale may also be one of the old analog types. I prefer a digital scale because it makes ounces easier to read and more accurate, however, for the sake of human weight loss, the accuracy of grams or ounces is not that critical. Use either one, but don't make it a daily habit of weighing yourself – it will be too easy to become influenced by the fluctuations.

Managing Hunger – Staying Full

The key to managing hunger is staying full, and the best way to stay full is to eat six small meals per day whenever possible. Don't wait till you're hungry; once you are hungry your appetite and sense of fullness will dictate how much you eat.

Since it takes at least fifteen minutes for the brain to register that the stomach is full, it's best to regulate your portions to specific sizes. Low fat snack bars that are low in sugar and fruits are a good way to maintain your hunger levels between meals.

I stay full by planning my main three years and using three snack periods in between, using fruit, celery/carrots packs and meal replacement bars for snacks.

The Psychology of Eating – Feeding Your Head

There is a psychology in the behavioral patterns in eating. Some are learned, some are genetic, but it's important to remember that reaching for something to eat can often be used as a way to medicate or deal with stressful life situations. Eating can also serve as an "oral fixation." These behaviors can be replaced with healthier ones.

Do you find yourself eating junk food in stressful situations? Many people do. Recognizing this behavior is the first step toward change. Once you identify a behavior, you should strive to reframe it into a healthier one. For instance, if you crave and like to eat chocolate candy bars when you are at work and a stressful meeting in coming up, instead of reaching for a Snickers bar or running down to the cafeteria for a similar fix like a cheese Danish or a doughnut, try having a low-sugar snack bar on hand.

It may not be the same fix as the real thing, but slowly you will come to accept the replacement as an ideal replacement, and the reinforcement of this behavior will be the weight loss and the empowerment you feel when you have overcome a major hurdle.

Our brains are supercomputers that simply respond to the programs (classical conditioning) we give them.

Stress and Anxiety – How to Cope

On the subject of stress and anxiety, there are other ways to cope other than reaching for comfort foods. An excellent way to combat stress is to use the "One Minute Relaxation Technique" explained later in this book, as well as deep breathing, exercise and yoga programs.

A daily routine that includes exercise, simple stretching, deep breathing, relaxation techniques and meditation can work wonders. These techniques do not require long hours each week to obtain results. Just a few minutes of each per day can make a real difference in your ability to beat stress, and as a result, eat less comfort foods.,

The Food Addiction Epidemic

We see evidence of food addiction everywhere in our society. The number of overweight Americans has skyrocketed in the past several decades, and the food industry is not our friend.

The fast food industry in particular not only provides us with a convenient drive-through fix for this addiction, they engineer their food products to fuel that addiction. Empty caloric and great-tasting foods served up by the fast food industry are scientifically designed to set up addictive cravings.

These addictions are set up from an early age, as we see at the fast food industry's marketing and advertising campaigns aimed at children. Tie-ins to popular age-oriented movies, superheroes and cartoon characters are no accident. Billions of dollars are spent each year on marketing to kids in order to set up food addictions that will carry many kids into adulthood and on into an early grave.

I had a college professor in my anatomy/physiology class that once said "most Americans dig their own graves with a spoon" and a truer adage has never been spoken.

About Food Addictions

Obsession and addiction to food can be similar to addiction to alcohol or drugs. Food addiction is a disease in which the addict craves refined sugar, flour and fats just as a cocaine addict craves cocaine. Food addicts get a feeling of pleasure and comfort from these foods and therefore continue to seek out the pleasure/comfort feelings. They use food to numb feelings of pain, anger, or depression. The food addict is often obsessed, unable to control the behavior even when they know intellectually of the negative health consequences. The physical craving overrides the power to make better eating decisions.

There are several types of food addictions:

Binge eating (compulsive overeating). The binge eater compulsively overeats and is unable to control their food intake. They often try to lose weight by dieting, but often gain back the initial weight loss, plus add more pounds. The binge eater eats when not physically hungry, often feels self-disgust and guilt, a cycle which can lead to depression and isolation. Their eating and weight gain can interfere with relationships, work, health and self-esteem.

Bulimia Nervosa is a potentially life-threatening disease in which the addict compulsively cycles between binge eating followed by attempts to prevent weight gain through purging behaviors. The Bulimic individual is often obsessed with body shape and weight, becomes withdrawn and secretive, feels guilt about their obsession, and may experience depression, irritability and severe mood swings.

Anorexia Nervosa is a progressive often-fatal disease in which the person is obsessed with controlling their food intake to maintain a thin body image. They often have a distorted view of their body image, seeing themselves as fat, even when they may look emaciated to others. A 15% or more below normal body weight is considered anorexic. Persons suffering from Anorexia often have difficulty eating in public, feel disgust towards food, yet play with or exhibit odd rituals around food. They have an intense fear of weight gain, may be obsessed with exercise, lies about food intake and becomes socially withdrawn. Their lack of food intake deprives the body of required nutrients and can lead to severe health problems and death.

Determining if someone is a food addict is not based on their weight, but rather the degree to which the behaviors towards food have caused deterioration in the quality of life and health. Food addiction can be treated. Diets and starvation are not the answer. Recovery from this devastating disease requires the person to deal with their feelings of anger, fear and depression, the feelings that are being numbed by the food substances.

Metabolism: How It Works and How To Work It

Metabolism is the natural rate at which your body burns fuel. Each person has their own unique metabolic rate, which is why some people can eat anything they want and never gain an ounce, while others can gain weight quite easily by eating very little.

Being aware of your metabolic rate and using it determines how much or how little or how much you can eat and approximately how much exercise or activity is required to maintain your ideal weight.

Why eating frequently increases metabolism

The more frequently you eat, the higher your metabolism will rise as your body steps up its fuel storage and burning to handle the excess calories. The less you eat, the slower your metabolism becomes, because the body naturally adjusts itself to storing food as fat as a survival mechanism.

One of the key elements to weight loss and weight balance is to eat times per day to keep your metabolic rate high. The good news is you don't have to go hungry to lose weight, and in fact, going hungry can actually sabotage your weight loss program.

WHAT TO EAT – AND HOW TO EAT IT

It's all about balancing protein, fat and carbohydrates. Depending on what your goals are, you can adjust the balance and percentages of each to accomplish your objective.

Carbohydrates

Carbohydrates are the body's primary source for fuel. With the exception of some isolated populations (such as the Inuits, who traditionally subsisted primarily on fats and proteins), carbohydrates comprise the majority of calories in most modern human diets.

Carbohydrates are found in a wide-range of foods including grains, breads, beans, nuts, milk, vegetables, fruits, cookies, sugar and soda. Because of their molecular structure, the body can break them down quickly and efficiently into glucose, which can be readily used by the body as energy.

Carbohydrates come in a variety of forms including sugars, starches and fiber. Depending on their structure, they may also fall into one of two groups: simple carbohydrates and complex carbohydrates.

Simple carbohydrates include sugars like sucrose (table sugar), fructose (fruit sugar) and "grape sugars" which are glucose or dextrose. Of the three, glucose and dextrose are the simplest forms and the carbohydrates most easily utilized by the body for energy since they are the most easily digested.

Complex carbohydrates contain three or more linked sugars, and thus require the body to work harder to break them down into glucose for energy. Some complex carbohydrates, like fruit or vegetable fibers, for example, cannot be broken down by the body and are passed through undigested.

Protein

Protein is made up of amino acids, which are the building blocks of all cells … and life.

Protein is used by the body to build, maintain and replace tissue (including muscle, hair, skin, organs and glands), as well as to produce hemoglobin, maintain proper immune function, and produce essential hormones and enzymes.

Protein can also be broken down into glucose (although not as efficiently as carbohydrates) for energy. Without protein, your body would be unable to build muscle and carry out many of its essential functions.

Foods that contain protein are broke into two groups: *complete proteins* and *incomplete proteins.*

Complete proteins contain all nine essential amino acids that the body cannot otherwise produce on its own. With the exception of soybeans, complete proteins are only found in animal foods like meat, poultry, fish, eggs, and milk and dairy products.

Incomplete proteins lack one or more of the nine essential amino acids. Incomplete sources of protein include most vegetables, as well as nuts, beans, seeds, peas and grains. Soybeans, however, are a complete protein.

Although vegetable sources of protein are incomplete, you can combine them to arrive at a complete protein. For example, by combining brown rice and beans, you get all nine essential amino acids. This is why it's even more critical for vegetarians or vegans to have carefully balanced meals when it comes to incorporating different sources of non-animal protein into their daily diet.

Also, while it is not necessary to consume all nine amino acids at the same time to meet your basic protein needs (the body can actually "pool" amino acids for later use), there may be benefits to consuming complete proteins at certain times of the day.

For example, having all nine essential amino acids available to the body immediately following an intensive workout may help with recovery and blunt catabolism (muscle breakdown.)

Protein is especially important for individuals who are engaged in intense physical activity or training, because it plays such an important role in the creation and repair of muscle and connective tissue. For those individuals, daily protein requirements may be greater than among the general population.

Fats

Like carbohydrates, fats have acquired something of a bad reputation, especially among dieters.

Part of this was fueled by research three decades ago that linked diets high in saturated fat with increased risk of heart disease and certain cancers, and part of it was the public's tendency to lump all fats together as "bad."

When food marketers jumped on the bandwagon in the 80s and began introducing "fat-free" foods, it seemed that everyone became obsessed with eating less fat, even if that meant eating more sugar and refined carbs than ever before.

However, fats are an essential macronutrient and some dietary fat is required for survival.

Indeed, the body needs fat to carry out a number of important processes. For example, some dietary fat is required to absorb certain fat-soluble vitamins such as vitamins A, D, E, K and caratanoids. Fat also plays a role in maintaining cell membranes, and people need some body fat to cushion their organs. The body even needs some cholesterol to produce certain key hormones, such as testosterone. Fat also is a concentrated form of energy, and when consumed with carbohydrates can slow their digestion and keep blood sugar levels stabilized.

More importantly, recent research has started to distinguish between the protective qualities of certain healthy fats, like the Omega 3 fatty acids contained in fish and flaxseed and monounsaturated fats from things like olive oil, from the "bad" fats like saturated and Trans fats. Indeed, some researchers are even questioning whether the original studies linking diets high in saturated fat with increased heart disease are as conclusive as originally thought.

Bottom line is that healthy fats from sources like olive oil, fish, avocados and nuts and seeds have a place in any fit person's diet. While it's still a good idea to avoid excessive saturated fats and Trans Fats (which ironically, were once considered "healthy" substitutes for saturated animal fats like lard or butter), going the "no-fat" route is probably a sure-fire ticket to a fatter mid-section. And you miss out on all of the protective benefits of healthy fats in the process.

Putting It All Together: What's the Right Mix of Carbs, Protein and Fats?

So now that you understand the role of each macronutrient, let's get back to that "balanced-meal" thing.

Balancing your carbohydrates, proteins and fats is really a matter of percentages. There are basic guidelines issued by the USDA around recommended daily intake for carbs, protein and fats, but each individual is different and the USDA recommendations are based on an average person consuming either 1500 or 2000 calories a day.

If you consume more calories because of your training regimen, your percentages may still fall within these guidelines, but your total grams of carbs, protein and fats will be higher than the average person.

The USDA recommendations also assumes average activity levels, which may not be appropriate for someone who is very active, is engaging in regular weight training, is an athlete or is training for a marathon or triathlon.

Also, some people find that they are more sensitive to carbs in terms of weight gain, and have better results managing their weight by customizing there macro-nutrient profile to emphasize slightly more protein or even fats in their overall diet.

The USDA recommends that 45%-65% of a person's daily calories come from carbohydrates, 10%-35% from protein and 20%-35% from fats. While the fat percentages may seem high, it's important to realize that fat has more calories per gram than carbohydrates or protein.

So while the percentage is high, the actual amount of fat that you consume under these guidelines is fairly low — typically less than 60 grams from a 2000-calorie diet.

Protein: How Much Is Enough for Fit People?

In terms of protein, there is debate over how much protein active individuals need each day — especially those engaging in weight or resistance training or athletic activities.

The USDA doesn't make a distinction between athletes and average people with lower activity levels when it comes to protein. The recommended minimum amount for men ages 19-70 is 46 grams of protein a day, and for women in the same age group, 46 grams of protein.

If you are performing intense weight training and are very active, your protein requirements may be significantly higher — anywhere from 0.8 grams per kg of bodyweight to 1-1.5 grams per kg of bodyweight.

While the USDA has not issued revised protein guidelines for individuals performing weight training or endurance exercises, there is a fairly convincing body of peer-reviewed research that does suggest higher protein consumption for people engaged in these types of activities. Those studies tended to look at protein consumption in excess of 1 gram per kg of bodyweight.

Again, it's important to remember that the total grams of protein that you consume are a percentage of your overall calories. So if you are eating 1800 calories a day, and 34% percent of them come from protein, you'll be consuming around 637 calories from protein, which is 159 grams of protein each day. While the absolute number may seem high, this is still within the US RDA guidelines. This is why absolute recommendations for how many grams of protein you should eat tend to under-estimate actual protein requirements.

Meal Planning:
How Can I Make Sure I'm Getting the Right Mix of Carbs, Protein and Fats?

While you can certainly track all of this right down to the percentages and grams in your food log or with a calorie counting program, it's not always very practical.

A good rule of thumb is to always include a complex carb, a protein and a healthy fat in every meal or snack.

For example, if your lunch were a turkey sandwich on whole wheat bread with lettuce and tomato and a half serving of almonds, you'd be at a mix of 37% carbs, 33% protein, and 30% fats. This is actually very close to Dr. Barry Sears Zone Diet ratio of 40:30:30, which in my personal experience is a good target to aim for, especially for someone who is trying to gain muscle and shed some fat.

Bottom line is that specific ratios can vary slightly, provided you are making good, solid choices about the kinds of carbohydrates and fats you are including along with your protein.

The main objective should be to always have each of the three macronutrients in each of your 5-6 small meals each day. This will ensure that you always have the critical nutrients available to your body, will stabilize blood sugar and prevent hunger pangs later in the day, and will discourage you from overeating and storing the excess calories as fat.

The Carbohydrate Debate: Is It Valid?

In recent years carbohydrates have gotten a bad rap. Part of this stems from the popularity of low-carb, high-fat diets like Atkins which encourage people to reduce carbs to extremely low levels, and part of it comes from emerging research around the health risks associated with the consumption of large amounts of simple, refined carbohydrates.

Carbohydrates themselves are not bad. They play an important role in nutrition, because they are a quick and efficient way to deliver energy to your cells, which can power your workouts and every day activities.

The key here is to preference complex carbs over simple carbs. Complex carbs are lower on the Glycemic index, and thus don't cause the quick spikes in blood sugar that simple, refined carbs do. These blood sugar spikes have been linked to increased risk for diabetes, metabolic syndrome, heart disease and obesity. There is also some evidence that high-Glycemic diets may also encourage certain types of cancer.

Good sources of complex carbohydrates include whole grains like oatmeal, brown rice, and whole wheat, as well as fresh vegetables and fruits.

The Glycemic Index: What It Is, How It Works

The Glycemic index, Glycemic index, or GI is a measure of the effects of carbohydrates on blood sugar levels.

Carbohydrates that break down quickly during digestion and release glucose rapidly into the bloodstream have a high GI; carbohydrates that break down more slowly, releasing glucose more gradually into the bloodstream, have a low GI.

The concept was developed by Dr. David J. Jenkins and colleagues in 1980–1981 at the University of Toronto in their research to find out which foods were best for people with diabetes.

A lower Glycemic index suggests slower rates of digestion and absorption of the foods' carbohydrates and may also indicate greater extraction from the liver and periphery of the products of carbohydrate digestion. A lower Glycemic response usually equates to lower insulin demand but not always, and may improve long-term blood glucose control and blood lipids.

The insulin index is also useful, as it provides a direct measure of the insulin response to a food.

The Glycemic index of a food is defined as the area under the two-hour blood glucose response curve (AUC) following the ingestion of a fixed portion of carbohydrate (usually 50 g). The AUC of the test food is divided by the AUC of the standard (either glucose or white bread, giving two different definitions) and multiplied by 100.

The average GI value is calculated from data collected in 10 human subjects. Both the standard and test food must contain an equal amount of available carbohydrate. The result gives a relative ranking for each tested food.[2]

The current validated methods use glucose as the reference food, giving it a Glycemic index value of 100 by definition.

This has the advantages of being universal and producing maximum GI values of approximately 100. White bread can also be used as a reference food, giving a different set of GI values (if white bread = 100, then glucose ≈ 140). For people whose staple carbohydrate source is white bread, this has the advantage of conveying directly whether replacement of the dietary staple with a different food would result in faster or slower blood glucose response. The disadvantages with this system are that the reference food is not well defined and the GI scale is culture dependent.

Your body performs best when your blood sugar is kept relatively constant. If your blood sugar drops too low, you become lethargic and/or experience increased hunger. And if it goes too high, your brain signals your pancreas to secrete more insulin.

Insulin brings your blood sugar back down, but primarily by converting the excess sugar to stored fat. Also, the greater the rate of increase in your blood sugar, the more chance that your body will release an excess amount of insulin, and drive your blood sugar back down too low.

Therefore, when you eat foods that cause a large and rapid Glycemic response, you may feel an initial elevation in energy and mood as your blood sugar rises, but this is followed by a cycle of increased fat storage, lethargy, and more hunger!

Although increased fat storage may sound bad enough, individuals with diabetes (diabetes mellitus, types 1 and 2) have an even worse problem. Their bodies inability to secrete or process insulin causes their blood sugar to rise too high, leading to a host of additional medical problems.

The theory behind the Glycemic Index is simply to minimize insulin-related problems by identifying and avoiding foods that have the greatest effect on your blood sugar.

For non-diabetics, there are times when a rapid increase in blood sugar (and the corresponding increase in insulin) may be desirable. For example, after strenuous physical activity, insulin also helps move glucose into muscle cells, where it aids tissue repair.

Because of this, some coaches and physical trainers recommend high-GI foods (such as sports drinks) immediately after exercise to speed recovery.

Also, it's not Glycemic Index alone that leads to the increase in blood sugar. Equally important is the amount of the food that you consume. The concept of Glycemic Index combined with total intake is referred to as "Glycemic Load", and is addressed in the next section...

My view of the Glycemic Index is that it's overly complicated, and that simple weight control gets right down to keeping an eye on good carbs and bad carbs.

It's easy to get carried away with charts, tables and indexes, but the simplified way to weight loss is to watch your portions, keep a healthy balance of proteins carbs and fats, and leave Glycemic index tables in the dust.

However, every person responds psychologically to different methods. If following the GI seems to speak to you in a unique way, and you are seeing results from using it, by all means do so.

Fast Food Solutions – What's Good In Fast Food?

Very little, it turns out. Fast food is engineered food: it's designed to be prepared quickly, not break down under prolonged periods under heat lamps, not be messy when eaten when on the move, and most importantly, to taste good and create a psychological and physiological craving to consume more.

There is not much value in the nutritional content of most fast foods, which tends to be high in fat, cholesterol and salt, and as such, is to be avoided whenever possible.

Most nutritionists will agree there is nothing wrong with indulging in your favorite burger or fries occasionally and in moderation, but making it a staple of your regular diet is what can lead to obesity and heart disease.

Many of us are on the run constantly. In our work environments, lunchtimes are also a short window and fast food shops beckon from every corner.

There are ways to use the convenience of the fast food chains to eat healthier.

McDonalds, for instance (as well as many of the chains) offer low calorie salads. One such example is the Grilled Chicken Caesar salad. (220 calories). Served with Newman's Own vinaigrette dressing (40 calories), this is a decent nutritional lunch item from a major fast food chain that weighs in at only 260 calories and 10 grams of fat.

Keep in mind, though, that the above item delivers 680 milligrams of sodium, and if you are on a salt-restricted diet, this must be considered in your recommended intake per day.

Salad items are usually your best bet when using the fast food chains, but make sure you consult the nutritional charts (available online, at each restaurant, and in the back of this book.)

Salads can contain ingredients that can send the caloric and fat count (not to mention sodium) soaring. The dressing is a particularly crafty culprit: stick with low calorie alternatives like vinaigrette, whenever possible.

Many fast food restaurants and convenience stores such as 7-11 are now offering fresh fruits for people on the run. If you find yourself unprepared and must use local convenience stores and fast food chains, go with salads and fresh fruits whenever possible.

A second alternative when using convenience stores are canned fruits: but make sure you drain off the heavy syrup if they come packaged as such.

An excellent source for learning the nutritional value and tasty alternatives to the national restaurant chain menus is a book called *"Eat This, Not That," by David Zinczenko and Matt Goulding.*

This wonderful resource book is a colorful and well-written study on "food swaps" you can make when eating at not only the fast food chains, but the national sit-down chains as well, and is highly recommended.

NOTE: The above authors also have two other guides that are quite helpful:

Eat This Not That! Supermarket Survival Guide: The No-Diet Weight Loss Solution

Cook This, Not That! The Kitchen Survival Guide

Frozen Foods

Contrary to some popular belief, foods that are frozen actually maintain their nutritional value, although it does slowly diminish over time. The thing to remember is that most prepared frozen food items are processed foods to begin with, i.e, they are loaded with sodium, preservatives and fat.

Preparing your own meals and freezing them is an excellent alternative to buying processed frozen foods, and is cheaper and much healthier for you.

However, processed frozen foods do offer benefits to those who have no time to cook, desire portion control and added nutrients (nutrients such as vitamins and minerals added during the preparation process.)

As always, there are many different degrees of quality in the ingredients used in different brands. For example, you may consider shopping for your frozen foods in a health food store that has a frozen food section.

Read the labels! Stay away from excessive fat, sodium and preservatives when selecting processed frozen foods. Which leads us to the subject of...

Processed Foods

Mass production of food is much cheaper overall than individual production of meals from raw ingredients. Therefore, a large profit potential exists for the manufacturers and suppliers of processed food products.

Individuals may see a benefit in convenience, but rarely see any direct financial cost benefit in using processed food as compared to home preparation. Poor quality ingredients and sometimes questionable processing and preservation methods detract greatly from the overall benefit gained by individual consumers.

More and more people live in the cities far away from where food is grown and produced. In many families the adults are working away from home and therefore there is little time for the preparation of food based on fresh ingredients.

The food industry offers products that fulfill many different needs: From peeled potatoes that only have to be boiled at home to fully prepared ready meals that can be heated up in the microwave oven within a few minutes.

Benefits of food processing include toxin removal, preservation, easing marketing and distribution tasks, and increasing food consistency.

In addition, it increases seasonal availability of many foods, enables transportation of delicate perishable foods across long distances, and makes many kinds of foods safe to eat by de-activating spoilage and pathogenic microorganisms.

Modern supermarkets would not be feasible without modern food processing techniques, long voyages would not be possible, and military campaigns would be significantly more difficult and costly to execute.

Modern food processing also improves the quality of life for people with allergies, diabetics, and other people who cannot consume some common food elements. Food processing can also add extra nutrients such as vitamins.

Processed foods are often less susceptible to early spoilage than fresh foods, and are better suited for long distance transportation from the source to the consumer. Fresh materials, such as fresh produce and raw meats, are more likely to harbor pathogenic micro-organisms (e.g. Salmonella) capable of causing serious illnesses.

In general, fresh food that has not been processed other than by washing and simple kitchen preparation, may be expected to contain a higher proportion of naturally-occurring vitamins, fiber and minerals than an equivalent product processed by the food industry. Vitamin C, for example, is destroyed by heat and therefore canned fruits have a lower content of vitamin C than fresh ones.

Food processing can lower the nutritional value of foods, and introduce hazards not encountered with naturally-occurring products.

Processed foods often include food additives, such as flavorings and texture-enhancing agents, which may have little or no nutritive value, or be unhealthy.

Preservatives added or created during processing to extend the 'shelf-life' of commercially-available products, such as nitrites or sulphites, may cause adverse health effects.

Use of low-cost ingredients that mimic the properties of natural ingredients (e.g. cheap chemically-hardened vegetable oils in place of more-expensive natural saturated fats or cold-pressed oils) have been shown to cause severe health problems, but are still in widespread use because of cost concerns and lack of consumer knowledge about the effects of substitute ingredients.

Processed foods often have a higher ratio of calories to other essential nutrients than unprocessed foods, a phenomenon referred to as "empty calories".

So-called junk food, produced to satisfy consumer demand for convenience and low cost, are most often mass-produced processed food products.

Again, read the labels as you shop and carefully plan your weekly diet regimen.

Sugar, Flour and Salt – The Hidden Poisons

Sugar

The average American consumes an astounding 2-3 pounds of sugar each week, which is not surprising considering that highly refined sugars in the forms of sucrose (table sugar), dextrose (corn sugar), and high-fructose corn syrup are being processed into so many foods such as bread, breakfast cereal, mayonnaise, peanut butter, ketchup, spaghetti sauce, and a plethora of microwave meals.

In the last 20 years, we have increased sugar consumption in the U.S. 26 pounds to 135 lbs. of sugar per person per year! Prior to the turn of this century (1887-1890), the average consumption was only 5 lbs. per person per year! Cardiovascular disease and cancer was virtually unknown in the early 1900's.

One of sugar's major drawbacks is that it raises the insulin level, which inhibits the release of growth hormones, which in turn depresses the immune system. This is not something you want to take place if you want to avoid disease.

An influx of sugar into the bloodstream upsets the body's blood-sugar balance, triggering the release of insulin, which the body uses to keep blood-sugar at a constant and safe level.

Insulin also promotes the storage of fat, so that when you eat sweets high in sugar, you're making way for rapid weight gain and elevated triglyceride levels, both of which have been linked to cardiovascular disease.

Complex carbohydrates tend to be absorbed more slowly, lessening the impact on blood-sugar levels.

Sugar Depresses The Immune System

We have known this for decades. It was only in the 1970's that researchers found out that vitamin C was needed by white blood cells so that they could phagocytes viruses and bacteria. White blood cells require a 50 times higher concentration inside the cell as outside so they have to accumulate vitamin C.

There is something called a "phagocyte index" which tells you how rapidly a particular macrophage or lymphocyte can gobble up a virus, bacteria, or cancer cell. It was in the 1970's that Linus Pauling realized that white blood cells need a high dose of vitamin C and that is when he came up with his theory that you need high doses of vitamin C to combat the common cold.

We know that glucose and vitamin C have similar chemical structures, so what happens when the sugar levels go up? They compete for one another upon entering the cells. And the thing that mediates the entry of glucose into the cells is the same thing that mediates the entry of vitamin C into the cells.

If there is more glucose around, there is going to be less vitamin C allowed into the cell. It doesn't take much: a blood sugar value of 120 reduces the phagocyte index by 75%. So when you eat sugar, think of your immune system slowing down to a crawl.

Here we are getting a little bit closer to the roots of disease. It doesn't matter what disease we are talking about, whether we are talking about a common cold or about cardiovascular disease, or cancer or osteoporosis, the root is always going to be at the cellular and molecular level, and more often than not insulin is going to have its hand in it, if not totally controlling it.

The health dangers which ingesting sugar on a habitual basis creates are certain. Simple sugars have been observed to aggravate asthma, move mood swings, provoke personality changes, muster mental illness, nourish nervous disorders, deliver diabetes, hurry heart disease, grow gallstones, hasten hypertension, and add arthritis.

Because refined dietary sugars lack minerals and vitamins, they must draw upon the body's micro-nutrient stores in order to be metabolized into the system. When these storehouses are depleted, destabilization of cholesterol and fatty acid is impeded, contributing to higher blood serum triglycerides, cholesterol, promoting obesity due to higher fatty acid storage around organs and in sub-cutaneous tissue folds.

Because sugar is devoid of minerals, vitamins, fiber, and has such a deteriorating effect on the endocrine system, major researchers and major health organizations (American Dietetic Association and American Diabetic Association) agree that sugar consumption in America is one of the 3 major causes of degenerative disease.

Honey Is A Simple Sugar

There are 4 classes of simple sugars which are regarded by most nutritionists as "harmful" to optimal health when prolonged consumption in amounts above 15% of the carbohydrate calories are ingested: Sucrose, fructose, honey, and malts.

Some of you may be surprised to find honey here. Although honey is a natural sweetener, it is considered a refined sugar because 96% of dry matter are simple sugars: fructose, glucose and sucrose.

It is little wonder that the honey bear is the only animal found in nature with a problem with tooth-decay (honey decays teeth faster than table sugar).

Honey has the highest calorie content of all sugars with 65 calories/tablespoon, compared to the 48 calories/tablespoon found in table sugar. The increased calories are bound to cause increased blood serum fatty acids, as well as weight gain, on top of the risk of more cavities.

Flour

Enriched flour is flour in which most of the natural vitamins and minerals have been extracted. This is done in order to give bread a finer texture, increase shelf life and prevent bugs from eating it (bugs will die if they attempt to live off it).

Why is enriched flour bad?

When the bran and the germ (the parts of the wheat that contain vitamins and minerals) are removed, your body absorbs wheat differently. Instead of being a slow, steady process through which you get steady bursts of energy, your body breaks down enriched flour too quickly, flooding the blood stream with too much sugar at once.

Your body then has to work hard to absorb the excess and stores it as fat. This causes quick highs and lows in your blood-sugar level which can lead to type-two diabetes and obesity.

All this and you're not even getting close to the amount of nutrients that whole grains contain.

Whole grains are richer in dietary fiber, antioxidants, protein (and in particular the amino acid lysine), dietary minerals (including magnesium, manganese, phosphorus, and selenium), and vitamins (including niacin, vitamin B6, and vitamin E).

By eating whole grains you reduce the risk of some forms of cancer, digestive system diseases, coronary heart disease, diabetes, and obesity.

There are many products that seem healthy on the front but in reality they are not. If the bread you are buying says "soft wheat" or "multi-grain" make sure you still read the ingredients.

Most of these breads are primarily made with enriched flour. Even if the word "enriched" is not there, if it does not say "whole" Avoid it. Don't get fooled by color either.

Even if it's brown, unbleached wheat flour is still missing the bran and the germ that contain essential nutrients as well as the fiber that aids digestion.

Look for products that say 100% whole wheat. Trader Joes carries spaghetti that is 100% whole wheat and tastes great.

Foods that commonly contain enriched flour

Bread
Pasta
Chicken nuggets (breaded)
Pizza
Pie crust
Crackers
Cake
Cookies
Brownies
Pretzels
Donuts

Sugar Cravings and Alternatives

Sugar has really no equal in terms of taste. There are many alternative sugar substitutes on the market, none of them really very good. Saccharine and Nutra-Sweet type of products such as Stevia leave an unpleasant aftertaste.

Honey is not a bad alternative, but it has a different taste than sugar and it has its own drawbacks.

What I try to do is use as little sugar as possible in coffee and as flavoring for foods.

Much of sugar craving is actually carbohydrate craving. One way to satisfy this is with a tablespoon of peanut butter.

"There are many reasons why we go for sweet things," according to Wendy Fries of Web MD, an adviser and writer to the medical profession.

"That appetite may be hardwired. Sweet is the first taste humans prefer from birth," says Christine Gerbstadt, MD, RD, a dietitian and American Dietetic Association (ADA) spokeswoman.

Carbohydrates stimulate the release of the feel-good brain chemical serotonin. Sugar is a carbohydrate, but carbohydrates come in other forms, too, such as whole grains, fruits, and vegetables.

The taste of sugar also releases endorphins that calm and relax us, and offer a natural "high," says Susan Moores, MS, RD, a registered dietitian and nutrition consultant in St. Paul, Minn.

Sweets just taste good, too. And that preference gets reinforced by rewarding ourselves with sweet treats, which can make you crave it even more. With that entire going for it, why wouldn't we crave sugar?

The problem comes not when we indulge in a sweet treat now and then, but when we over-consume, something that's easy to do when sugar is added to many processed foods, including breads, yogurt, juices, and sauces.

And Americans do over-consume, averaging about 22 teaspoons of added sugars per day, according to the American Heart Association, which recommends limiting added sugars to about 6 teaspoons per day for women and 9 for men.

How to Stop Sugar Cravings: 8 Tips to Use Right Now

If you're craving sugar, here are some ways to tame those cravings.

Give in a little.

Eat a bit of what you're craving, maybe a small cookie or a fun-size candy bar, suggests Kerry Neville, MS, RD, a registered dietitian and ADA spokeswoman.

Enjoying a little of what you love can help you steer clear of feeling denied. Try to stick to a 150-calorie threshold, Neville says.

Combine foods.

If the idea of stopping at a cookie or a baby candy bar seems impossible, you can still fill yourself up and satisfy a sugar craving, too. "I like combining the craving food with a healthful one," Neville says. "I love chocolate, for example, so sometimes I'll dip a banana in chocolate sauce and that gives me what I'm craving, or I mix some almonds with chocolate chips." As a beneficial bonus, you'll satisfy a craving and get healthy nutrients from those good-for-you foods.

Go cold turkey.

Cutting out all simple sugars works for some people, although "the initial 48 to 72 hours are tough," Gerbstadt says. Some people find that going cold turkey helps their cravings diminish after a few days; others find they may still crave sugar but over time are able to train their taste buds to be satisfied with less.

Grab some gum.

If you want to avoid giving in to a sugar craving completely, try chewing a stick of gum, says nutrition advisor Dave Grotto, RD, LDN. "Research has shown that chewing gum can reduce food cravings," Grotto says.

Reach for fruit.

Keep fruit handy for when sugar cravings hit. You'll get fiber and nutrients along with some sweetness. And stock up on foods like nuts, seeds, and dried fruits, says certified addiction specialist Judy Chambers, LCSW, CAS.

"Have them handy so you reach for them instead of reaching for the old [sugary] something."

Get up and go.

When a sugar craving hits, walk away. "Take a walk around the block or [do] something to change the scenery," to take your mind off the food you're craving, Neville suggests.

Choose quality over quantity.

"If you need a sugar splurge, pick a wonderful, decadent sugary food," Moores says. But keep it small. For example, choose a perfect dark chocolate truffle instead of a king-sized candy bar, then "savor every bite – slowly," Moores says.

Grotto agrees. "Don't swear off favorites – you'll only come back for greater portions. Learn to incorporate small amounts in the diet but concentrate on filling your stomach with less sugary and [healthier] options."

Eat regularly.

Waiting too long between meals may set you up to choose sugary, fatty foods that cut your hunger, Moores says. Instead, eating every three to five hours can help keep blood sugar stable and help you "avoid irrational eating behavior," Grotto says. Your best bets? "Choose protein, fiber-rich foods like whole grains and produce," Moores says.

But won't eating more often mean overeating? Not if you follow Neville's advice to break up your meals. For instance, have part of your breakfast – a slice of toast with peanut butter, perhaps – and save some yogurt for a mid-morning snack. "Break up lunch the same way to help avoid a mid-afternoon slump," Neville says

How to Stop Sugar Cravings: 5 Tips for the Long Term

One of the best ways to manage sugar cravings is to stop them before they start. To help you do that:

Skip artificial sweeteners.

Artificial sweeteners may sound like a great idea, but "they don't lessen cravings for sugar and haven't demonstrated a positive effect on our obesity epidemic," says Grotto, author of 101 Foods That Could Save Your Life.

Reward yourself for successfully managing sugar cravings.

Your reward could be large or small. Remember why you're working on it and then reward yourself for each successful step.

Slow down.

For one week, focus on your sugar cravings and think about what you're eating, suggests Chambers. Diet mayhem often results from lack of planning. So slow down, plan, "and eat what you intend to eat, instead of eating when you're desperate," Chambers says.

Get support.

Many people turn to sweet foods when they're stressed, depressed, or angry. But food doesn't solve emotional issues. Consider whether emotions are involved in your sugar cravings and whether you need help to find other solutions to those emotional problems.

Mix it up.

You may need more than one strategy to thwart sugar cravings. One week you may find success with one tactic, and another week calls for an alternative approach. What's important is to "have a 'bag of tricks' to try," Gerbstadt tells WebMD. To tame sugar cravings, you really need to "figure out what works for you," Neville says.

Lastly, go easy on yourself.

It may take time to get a handle on your sugar cravings. "It's difficult to shift any system – whether it's the world economy or your eating," Chambers says.

Flaxseed Oil – Benefits and Beyond

Flaxseed is the seed of the flax plant, which is believed to have originated in Egypt. It grows throughout Canada and the northwestern United States.

Not surprisingly, flaxseed oil comes from flaxseeds.

Flaxseed is most commonly used as a laxative, but is also used for hot flashes and breast pain. Flaxseed oil is used for different conditions than flaxseed, including arthritis. Both flaxseed and flaxseed oil have been used for high cholesterol levels and in an effort to prevent cancer.

Whole or crushed flaxseed can be mixed with water or juice and taken by mouth. Flaxseed is also available in powder form.

Flaxseed oil is available in liquid and capsule form. Flaxseed contains lignans (phytoestrogens, or plant estrogens), while flaxseed oil preparations lack lignans.

Flaxseed contains soluble fiber, like that found in oat bran, and may have a laxative effect.

Studies of flaxseed preparations to lower cholesterol levels report mixed results. A 2009 review of the clinical research found that cholesterol-lowering effects were more apparent in postmenopausal women and in people with high initial cholesterol concentrations.

Some studies suggest that alpha-linolenic acid (a substance found in flaxseed and flaxseed oil) may benefit people with heart disease. But not enough reliable data are available to determine whether flaxseed is effective for heart conditions.

Study results are mixed on whether flaxseed decreases hot flashes.

Although some population studies suggest that flaxseed might reduce the risk of certain cancers, there is not enough research to support a recommendation for this use.

NCCAM is funding studies on flaxseed. Recent studies are looking at its potential role in preventing or treating arteriosclerosis (hardening of the arteries), breast cancer, and ovarian cysts.

Side Effects and Cautions

Flaxseed and flaxseed oil supplements seem to be well tolerated. Few side effects have been reported.

Flaxseed, like any supplemental fiber source, should be taken with plenty of water; otherwise, it could worsen constipation or, in rare cases, even cause intestinal blockage. Both flaxseed and flaxseed oil can cause diarrhea.

The fiber in flaxseed may lower the body's ability to absorb medications that are taken by mouth.

Flaxseed should not be taken at the same time as any conventional oral medications or other dietary supplements.

Both fish oil and flax seed oil have benefits and potential drawbacks. Fish oil is an excellent and usually uncontaminated source of EPA and DHA, which the body uses to make the "calming" omega-3 fatty acids and keep the brain healthy.

Consuming them directly can ensure that one gets enough.

Flax seed oil contains ALA, which the body can use to make all the omega-3s that it needs. The body needs ALA to make other omega-3s, even when it gets enough EPA and DHA from fish or fish oils.

As for drawbacks, some fish oil products are contaminated, and even those that are not may have undergone a cleaning process that creates a small percentage of toxic molecules. On the other hand, getting all one's omega-3s from flax oil means that one needs to consume significantly more.

Also, it is possible to ingest too much omega-3s, even though the greater health risk is of consuming too much omega-6 LA. Also, people with congestive heart failure should take omega-3s only with the full knowledge and active supervision of their physician.

In conclusion, why limit oneself to either/or when it's better to have both/and? Eating a modest amount of fish or fish oil (or algae-based DHA supplements) ensures a direct supply of EPA and DHA, while adding flax seed oil to one's diet ensures a healthy intake level of ALA. Every cell in your body will thank you for it.

Vitamins and Minerals – The Easy Way

The recommended daily intake, or RDA, of most vitamins and minerals was established about 60 years ago and is beyond antiquated. And, it only addresses vitamin deficiency symptoms, not their optimal intake for health, and it is frequently based on inadequate studies:

Did you know that the recommendation of 60 mg a day of vitamin C is based on a questionable study of six prisoners, conducted in the late 1940s?

This recommendation has only recently been revised, when the Institute of Medicine proposed increasing the recommended daily intake it to 90 mg., which insures that this change has no real health benefit to anyone.

So, how much vitamin C do we need to stay healthy?

A well-designed study conducted in 1996 by the National Institute of Health recommended at least 220 mg of vitamin C a day for young men consuming ideal diets. But what about older people, cigarette smokers, those who have to cope with stress, who live in polluted urban areas, or suffer from diseases? For people who fall into these categories the demands for vitamin C increase tremendously.

Health authorities recommend that zoo monkeys, whom, like humans, cannot produce their own vitamin C, need about 900 mg supplemented in their diets.

We should be more concerned with vitamin insufficiency, than with over-consumption.

According to the 2nd National Health and Nutrition Examination Survey, in the US, a country with high economic levels and nutrition awareness, between 50%-80% of people consume less than official recommendation of vitamins C, E, A, and D. The standards for the official recommendations of these vitamins is very low, to start with.

Studies repeatedly confirm that our diets are largely deficient in folic acid, B vitamins, niacin, zinc, calcium, and many other nutrients. So, instead of eliminating basic nutrient deficiencies, we are being confused with ostensible problems of vitamin excess.

However, we need vitamins and, we often need them in doses that are higher than currently recommended by the authorities.

Even very large doses of vitamins are generally safe. These nutrients are already contained in our bodies and they need to be constantly replenished.

They are naturally absorbed so our bodies will use what they need and discard the rest. In case of vitamin C there have been almost a dozen recently published placebo-controlled, double-blind studies showing no adverse effects in people who take even 10 g of this nutrient for several years.

Many cancer patients were taking 150-200 g, which is 150,000 to 200,000 mg of vitamin C a day by IV injections, without any evidence of toxicity. In fact, the results were just the opposite, these doses were helpful in curing the spread of cancer in the body.

Also, other vitamins such as B vitamins, which our body needs primarily for various energy generating processes, are safe in a wide dosage range. The review of scientific research on this subject published by Dr. Bendich in the Annals of the New York Academy of Sciences concluded that there were no adverse reactions from taking 3 mg of vitamin B12 (this is about 1800 times the current official recommendation), vitamin B6 up to 500 mg (250 times the recommended level), vitamin B2 taken at daily doses of 200 mg (which is about 130 times higher than the recommended intake) and B1 (about 35 times the recommended RDA).

Many people, perhaps you as well, take supplemental vitamin B3, also known as nicotinic acid, for a natural control of their cholesterol levels. Some of those who took a large dose at once might have experienced a transient feeling of a hot flash. This reaction can be avoided if the vitamin dose is increased gradually or if vitamin B3 is taken in the form of niacinimide. In general, nicotinic acid can be taken in doses that exceed 50-150 times the official recommendation without any adverse effects.

Even vitamins that are not quickly eliminated by the body, such as fat-soluble vitamins A, D, E, and K, are safe in large doses.

For example, vitamin A, which is essential for vision, growth and repair of the body tissues, has beneficial effects when taken in doses about 5,000 to 10,000 IU a day. Its daily intake was tested in doses higher than that in people with specific health problems. In our body, vitamin A is produced from another nutrient, beta-carotene, which is a yellow pigment of fruits and vegetables. If we take beta-carotene, our body automatically converts it into the quantity of vitamin A it needs and eliminates the excess.

Another fat-soluble vitamin, Vitamin E, has health benefits when taken at daily doses exceeding our current RDAs. Not only is vitamin E safe at high intake levels, but there are no known adverse reactions even at doses of 3000 IU or higher, for prolonged periods. This is more than 200 times the official recommendation. When it is consumed at high doses, health benefits to heart disease, diabetes and other problems become apparent. But it is impossible to obtain such high amounts from diet alone, vitamin supplements are absolutely necessary.

Because of inadequate training at medical schools, many doctors look at vitamins as individual substances just as they look at pharmaceutical drugs.

However, in our body, vitamins work as a team and they cooperate with each other for a maximum effect. For instance, you do not need to take extreme amounts of vitamin E if you take vitamin C as well.

Vitamin C can recycle vitamin E in the body, compensating for its inadequate intake. It also cooperates with other nutrients, such as antioxidants lipoid acid and glutathione, vitamin B3 and coenzyme Q10.

New information about ostensible vitamin danger is promoted very quickly and becomes commonly accepted without any substantial evidence. A typical example is the popular conception that vitamin C causes kidney stones. Nearly every physician is aware of this "fact," but where is the evidence for it?

Several articles written have spread this myth. But when I looked up the references for the real source of this information, they directed me to books, letters, but not to any reputable clinical data. The citations in the books referred again to the same sources and to other books. So one author makes a statement and cites another author who did the same.

But what is the actual evidence? Three case control studies did not show any association between vitamin C and kidney stones. Another study conducted in 1997 on 45,000 men showed that those consuming 1.5 g, of vitamin C a day actually had a lower frequency of kidney stones than those who took only 250 mg of this vitamin A study published last year by

Harvard University researchers on 85,000 women also concluded that there is a lack of correlation between vitamin C intake and kidney stones.

The easy way to get your daily requirements of vitamins and minerals is to eat a balanced diet, and take a regular multi-vitamin supplement, which also provides your daily required intake of minerals.

In addition, your blood work may indicate a deficiency in certain elements, such as iron, in which case you should take an additional iron supplement.

If you are subject to easily bruise, for instance, or you are healing from an injury, it is recommended you take extra doses of vitamin C.

Calorie Counting

If cutting portions and watching what you eat does not seem to be getting you the desired results, you may need to start counting calories for everything you eat, and regulate your intake.

Food charts listing most foods and the food groups, and their caloric content are available online listed in the resources section of this book.

Use them to determine how many calories are contained in the foods you enjoy and regulate accordingly. Science tells us that 1 pound of fat is equal to 3500 calories, so a daily calorie deficit of 500 should result in 1 pound per week fat loss. In reality things don't quite work that efficiently!

Always try to aim for the "Fat Loss" daily calorie level.

The "Extreme Fat Loss" level is effectively a rock bottom calorie level. Do not attempt to immediately drop your calories to this level hoping for the quick fix - this may ultimately backfire. The Extreme Fat Loss level is listed to show the lowest calorie amount that could be considered. It should be seen as the exception rather than the rule.

It truly is better to burn the fat than to starve it.

The Weight Loss Plateau

Over time our bodies adapt to the lowered calorie level. Our body becomes more efficient at using energy (lowered metabolism), and therefore burns less fat.

This is why most of us reach a weight loss plateau. At this point, the only option is to boost metabolism; increased cardio, weight training, 'cheat' meals (i.e. occasional high-calorie meals), cycling (or zigzagging) calories, and even manipulating macro-nutrient ratios can all help to do this (don't forget adequate sleep and hydration). You often find that the nearer you get to your goal weight (or body fat percentage) - the harder things get!

Continually dropping calories only serves to lower metabolism even further - the moment you return to 'normal' eating - the weight comes back on.

Minimum Daily Calorie intake

It is difficult to set absolute bottom calorie levels, because everyone has different body composition and activity levels.

Health authorities do set some baselines - these are 1200 calories per day for women, and 1800 calories per day for men. This doesn't really make too much sense - are you are sedentary person with little muscle mass? Or someone who is tall, muscular, and exercises a lot? Absolute levels don't work - but do give us a starting point.

When reducing calories:

Try not to lower your calorie intake by more than 1000 calories below maintenance. Doing so may invoke the body's starvation response, which can lead to the Yo-yo dieting effect.

Try to gradually lower calories. A sudden drop (such as 500 calories or more) can cause your metabolism to slow.

What happens when calories are too low?

1) Muscle mass is broken down for energy (catabolism).

2) Metabolic rate will begin to drop (typically) after 3 days of very low calories - this is related to, and compounded by the loss of muscle mass.

3) With very low calories you risk sluggishness, nutritional deficiencies, fatigue, and often irritability. You are completely set-up for a regain in fat if you suddenly return to your previous eating patterns.

Lose Fat And Build Muscle?

Depending on your body type, it can be a very difficult balance trying to eat to burn fat, but retain or even build muscle. It's worth reading Tom Venuto's Burn the fat, feed the muscle

(BFFM) for valuable insight on how to balance this. But realize that there is no single answer for everyone. It is a process of trial and error - but you need a starting point.

The Half Portion Principle

An excellent and effective way to reduce your intake and lose weight is the half-portion principle. Whether you are eating on the run or at home, even in a restaurant, simply cut your portion in half.

This is easily done if you are dining in a restaurant with someone else – you can split one meal – and you save money!

I know may couples who have gone to fast food restaurants and cut a Big Mac in half and split the fries – it's a wonderful way to satisfy that fast food craving and save money to boot!

This also works with deserts too – try it!

Doubling Up:
Finding A Workmate To Team With

If you know of a friend, partner or family member interested in losing weight, you may consider teaming up with them and meeting regularly to compare notes.

Even a co-worker or classmate can be incredibly supportive and keep you grounded and keep temptation at bay.

There are also many weight-loss support groups both in your local community and online. Hooking up with these social networking groups allows you to stay on track, share your success stories, and make new friends.

Eating At Work

Many times our workday is filled with tension and stress. With hard work looming and time at a premium, it's all too easy to fall into the snack trap of eating the wrong things at the wrong times, and very often too much of them.

Simple planning is the key, for if you fail to plan you will plan to fail. One weekly trip to your grocery or health food store should supply you with everything you need to implement and maintain a successful weight maintenance program.

Eating at work is as simple as bringing a small cloth-insulated cooler (sold online or at any Target, Kmart or Wal-Mart store) with cut carrot and celery sticks, apples and/or other fruits to go; pre-made sandwiches, wraps or other low-calorie items.

Bring your lunch – salads are great. Avoid the takeout lunches served in the work cafeteria or local fast food.

Trader Joe's offers a great many pre-made sandwiches and wraps, or better yet you can prepare them in only a few minutes in the morning before you leave for work.

Wraps are wonderful foods – they can be made with whole wheat or natural tortillas, tomatoes, lettuce, sliced turkey and even a low-cal cheese slice.

(I personally don't like low-cal cheese – I put one slice of cheddar on mine and figure it into my daily caloric allocation.)

Office Dining: A Few Tips

Whatever you were eating at work, you have company: Recent studies, including two from the American Dietetic Association, show that more than a third of office workers are eating breakfast alongside their keyboards; as many as two-thirds regularly munch on lunch in their work offices; nine in 10 snack on the job; and 7 percent are even eating dinner desk-side.

Corporate America seems to be turning into a giant kitchen, where eating on the job has become a necessity for the time-crunched and stressed. The average "lunch hour" has shrunk to 36 minutes–and chocolate has become a bottom-drawer staple (its feel-good endorphins make tension easier to handle). But the number one reason for desk-side eating is hunger.

"Most office food isn't satisfying," says Baltimore nutritionist Colleen Pierre, RD. "Doughnuts, coffee, pastries, and candy give you temporary energy, but you're hungry a few hours later." It doesn't take long for the quick work fix to become a pattern. So Prevention tried an intervention.

First, we found volunteers at four work sites who let us rummage through their desks, briefcases, office kitchens, and coat pockets, leaving no crumb uninspected.

Then Pierre gave the volunteers an office makeover–a corporate downsizing, if you will. Here's her analysis and habit-breaking eating strategies.

The Group Nosh
The Haystack Group, Marietta, GA

Resumé: "A sweet tooth is a job requirement here," admits Stefanie Long, director of public relations, who shares this consumer research office with six others. Not a single one is on a diet, and all enjoy the same kinds of food. "When we chow down, we do it together. It's a social experience," says Holly Cline, an account manager.

Desk-Side Dining: Most of the work crew eat breakfast and lunch at the office. Once a week, the company's founder, Bonnie Ulman, brings in a baker's dozen of mini Cheddar muffins. "I believe in taking care of the staff," she says. Other days might begin with eating takeout Chick-fil-A Chicken Biscuits (buttermilk biscuits with a fried chicken patty) or bagels and cream cheese.

"Despite the fact that the coffeemaker is going all day and we just got an espresso machine, one of us goes to Starbucks–sometimes twice a day–with an office order for tall mochas, lattes, and hot apple ciders," reports Cline. On stressful days, she says, they drink larger, 16-ounce cups of their caffeinated drink of choice with an extra shot of espresso.

At least three times a week the group returns to Chick-fil-A for lunch, bringing back fried chicken sandwiches, fries, and Cokes. Alternatively, they might hit Taco Bell for Zesty Chicken Borders Bowls and an occasional Nachos Supreme. Or they'll go for chips and sandwiches from a nearby deli. Occasionally, they organize a potluck lunch. "At the last one, the chocolate-covered strawberries were the biggest hit," recalls Long.

Between the sugar and caffeine highs and lows, the entire office usually slumps around 3 pm. Their solution: chocolate. Last fall, to celebrate the completion of a book Ulman wrote, the group enjoyed eating two 3-pound bags of M&Ms and a pound each of Hershey's Kisses, candy corn, and candy pumpkins. After 3 days, only a handful of Kisses remained at work. "Once someone brought in apples, but they rotted in the fridge," says Cline.

"Work is the place to be bad," says Long. "No one here judges anyone. When you mention to someone that you ate half a bag of Oreos, they tell you it's okay because they did, too."

Office Overhaul Pierre says: Everyone should agree to have a breakfast that delivers more nutrients and fiber in fewer calories than chicken biscuits, muffins, or bagels with cream cheese. The caffeine in all that coffee is increasing everyone's stress hormones. Reaching for candy is a natural response and, because chocolate is also a stimulant, it fuels hunger.

Ulman would do everyone a favor by passing up the Cheddar muffins and bringing in a fruit basket to put near the printer or wherever people gather.

For lunch, cut back the fast-food trips to once or twice a week–and make better choices at the restaurants. At Taco Bell, for instance, the Bean Burrito has about half the calories and a third the saturated fat of the Zesty Chicken Border Bowl plus dressing.

On the remaining days, try the soup and salad bar at a nearby supermarket or organize a weekly potluck lunch and limit desserts to fruit.

If the Starbucks trips give people a much-needed break, skip anything topped with whipped cream and go for the steamed cider (180 calories) or decaffeinated, fat-free lattes (120 calories plus 35 percent of the calcium DV).

The Out-of-Balance Eater
Amy Brown, Chatsworth, CA

Resumé: This 37-year-old mom and public relations manager/editor for a corporate communications firm starts her day at 5 am, when she shares a breakfast of raisin bread with her toddler daughter. Brown leaves the house by 6, is in the office by 7, and works through lunch, eating her midday meal at her desk so she can head home by 4:40 pm.

"I do most of my eating at work," she says. "I cook dinner for my family, and have an artichoke myself because I'm too full from what I ate at the office."

Desk-Side Dining: "When I get to work, I usually take a scone or muffin from a tray that someone brings in for morning meetings," says Brown. When there are no pastries, she reaches into her desk drawer for her stash of almonds and crackers. Brown also keeps salad ingredients in the office fridge.

To complete her lunch, she brings in chicken, barbecued salmon, or other leftovers from the previous night's dinner. Once or twice a week, she gets a salad from a gourmet grocery store along with a cookie or brownie. "I have two or three sweet snacks a day," admits Brown, who often raids a bowl of peanut M&Ms in the office conference room.

Office Overhaul Pierre advises Brown: Stop starving yourself of real food. You eat a lot of desserts, but no balanced meals. Improve your poor eating at work habits and set a good example for your daughter by having breakfast and dinner with her, and eating the foods you want her to enjoy.

Unsweetened instant oatmeal (with a little honey, if you need some sweetener), milk, and fruit are fast and filling. Stir some chopped nuts into yours, too. The fiber in the cereal and fruit, and the protein in the nuts, will help keep you satisfied for several hours, so you won't need that scone. For a mid-morning snack, keep your favorite low-fat yogurt in the fridge for a good dose of calcium and to quell your cravings for sweets.

Bringing lunch from home is a great idea, but your salad needs to be bulked up in fat or protein to keep you full throughout the afternoon. Also, if you choose chicken instead of leftover salmon or another oily fish in the salad, be sure to use an olive oil-based vinaigrette or sprinkle on some nuts. For fiber, have a small whole-grain roll.

Instead of multi-tasking, give yourself 15 to 20 minutes to concentrate on your meal. You'll feel more relaxed and satisfied, and therefore less tempted later by peanut M&Ms. By dinnertime you'll be hungry enough to enjoy a meal with your family. Keep dried fruit in your desk drawer and fresh fruit in the fridge for a mid-afternoon snack.

The One-Track Snacker
Vickie Spang, Los Angeles

Resumé: The consummate professional, Spang, 53 and single and a chief marketing officer for a law firm, often works long hours. She tends to skip dinner unless she's invited out because it's too much trouble to cook for herself at the end of the day. "If I'm really hungry, I'll microwave a bag of popcorn when I get home."

Desk-Side Dining: Spang stashes Skippy Super Chunk Peanut Butter in her desk drawer (there's another jar in her car and one in her apartment). She helps herself to a heaping teaspoon for breakfast, another before lunch, and possibly another, later in the work day, if she works late.

Come lunchtime, Spang turns the counter at California Pizza Kitchen into another office. While she's eating her usual-tortilla soup and barbecued chicken salad with extra sauce-she does her reading. "I sit at the counter, read The Wall Street Journal, and open interoffice mail," she says.

Spang mostly drinks bottled water, but on an occasional morning, she'll have a V8 before work. "I don't like vegetables much, so this helps," she says. One thing you won't find in her office: a candy dish. "I read in a professional magazine that it sends the wrong signal; you seem more like a mom than a professional," she says.

Office Overhaul Pierre tells Spang: You need to start your work day with something nutritious and satisfying. Try a low-fat yogurt, drinkable yogurt, or a piece of string cheese with a few whole-grain crackers or a small whole-grain roll.

At lunchtime, since you're going to California Pizza Kitchen, how about eating pizza once in awhile? Or pasta? Or a sandwich? You don't eat much food at home, so your on-the-job meals need more variety and have to provide more of the fruits and vegetables that you need every day.

Some dishes to try: Vegetarian Pizza with Japanese Eggplant (any kid will tell you that veggies taste better when they're covered with cheese), Broccoli and Sun-Dried Tomato Fusilli, or the Grilled Rosemary Chicken Sandwich (stuffed with tomatoes and romaine lettuce).

Peanut butter is one of the best foods to keep in your desk. But instead of eating it plain, spread some on a banana, apple, celery stalk, or carrot. Pick up ready-to-eat baby carrots or apple slices (sold in a bag of five small packages), and prewashed and precut celery sticks. To get more grains, stash some whole-grain crackers in your work desk to eat plain or with peanut butter.

Finally, eat something for dinner if you're working late, or have a late-afternoon snack if you're planning to skip dinner at home. You could reheat your leftovers from California Pizza Kitchen or buy frozen meals (Tesoros makes a great Penne Toscana and a Chipotle de Azteca–rice with creamy pepper sauce plus grilled chicken, corn, and onions). Or have a bowl of whole-grain cereal with milk and berries. Smart, late-in-the-day snacks include the Athenos Traveler (hummus and pita bread packaged together), a premade fruit smoothie, and a package of sunflower seeds.

The Dorm-Style Diner
Lindsay Morgan, Denver

Resumé: A 30-year-old newlywed and director of community affairs for a university, Morgan recognizes that she rarely eats healthy foods in or out of the office. "I make a resolution, try it for 2 days, and then forget about it for 3 months," she says. Why? "I'm happy with my weight. I get good checkup reports from the doctor, and I play in a softball league," she explains. "I want to do better, but I can't get myself motivated."

Desk-Side Dining: Morgan starts her work day at the office with two cups of coffee with cream and Sweet'N Low. Three times a week, she brown-bags her lunch–often a turkey sandwich with chips or Goldfish crackers, and a can of cola. On the remaining days, she goes to Chipotle Mexican Grill, where she typically orders a chicken burrito with cheese, sour cream, and black beans, washing it down with a cola.

In the middle of the afternoon, she reaches into her desk drawer for a family-size package of Wonka Runts or Gobstoppers, hard candies that have been favorites since childhood. She's also fond of microwave popcorn. "Sometimes I polish off the whole bag for dinner when I work late," she says.

Office Overhaul Pierre advises Morgan: You're eating like a college student–skipping meals, drinking sodas, and noshing on chips, popcorn, and candy. You may be happy with your weight and health now, but this high-calorie, low-nutrient eating pattern will catch up with you. Instead of trying to make several changes at once and failing, choose one improvement and practice it for a month. That's about how long it takes for a new behavior to become a habit.

Start before you get to work with a breakfast that will keep you satisfied and energized. Try peanut butter on a whole-wheat English muffin, or a frozen whole-grain waffle, toasted and topped with yogurt and fruit. Once you get adjusted to that pattern, work on lunch.

Exchange your Goldfish and potato chips for a palmful of smoked almonds. Their healthy fats will sustain you throughout the afternoon. Next, bring in a piece of fruit to have after lunch.

Finally, try to cut back on your caffeine. Begin by replacing the cola with bottled water. Miss the bubbles? Try mineral water. Gradually decrease the coffee; replace one cup with decaffeinated green tea for the antioxidants.

While you're making these changes, buy a few more items for eating at work. Next to your candy, keep an assortment of dried fruits so sweets aren't your only option.

Also stash a StarKist Lunch To-Go kit (which includes tuna, mayo, relish, spoon, crackers, and even a mint) in your drawer for nights when you're working late. Another alternative: Store an Uncle Ben's Rice or Noodle Bowl in the office freezer.

Secrets to Smart Snacking

Snacking sometimes gets a bad rap, but snacking can be great for you when you choose sensible portions of nutritious snacks.

For instance, snacks can: Add good nutrition to your eating plan by providing important nutrients and filling in food groups you missed at meals.

- Give you fuel to keep going through the day.

- Dampen your appetite so you're less likely to overeat at meals.

Try these secrets to make the most of your snacks:

Follow the five food groups

Choose foods that contribute to the recommended daily food group amounts in your MyPyramid eating plan. For example:
- Whole-grain cereal, whole-grain crackers and popcorn from the Grains Group

- Broccoli florets, celery sticks and radishes from the Vegetables Group
- Apples, strawberries and raisins from the Fruit Group
- Reduced-fat cheese sticks and low fat or fat free yogurt from the Milk Group
- Nuts, sunflower seeds and hummus from the Meat & Beans Group

Make snacks part of the plan

Include snacks as part of your eating plan, not as "extras" or you might get too many calories.

Think about what food groups you're missing and use snacks to fill in the gaps. For instance, if you didn't have milk in the morning, snack on a serving of cheese or yogurt in the afternoon.

If you missed fruit during the day, snack on an orange or a banana in the evening.

Prepare to snack

Put nutritious snacks on your shopping list so you have plenty of nutritious options on hand.

Practice portion control

A smart snack is big enough to take the edge off your appetite, but not so big that you eat too many calories.

To control portions, use the serving size information on the Nutrition Facts label as a guide, put a portion of your snack on a plate or in a bowl rather than eating out of the bag or container, or choose snacks with built-in portion control such as NABISCO 100 CALORIE PACKS. For many people, a snack with 100 to 200 calories is about right.

Pack a snack

Toss a bag of baby carrots, a yogurt cup or some grapes in your lunch bag to stow in the office fridge for an afternoon snack. If you're on the go all day, bring along non-perishable items such as whole-wheat pretzels, nuts or dried fruit.

Choose vending machine snacks such as cereal bars, yogurt cups, small bags of nuts or trail mix, fresh fruit, fat free milk or 100% fruit juice. At the drive through, look for small green salads or fruit salads, bags or cups of fruit, or small cups or cones of low fat frozen yogurt or reduced-fat ice cream.

Time it right

Snack two or three hours before your next meal to take the edge off your hunger. You might be less likely to munch while you make dinner or overeat at your meal.

Skip distracted snacking

Break the habit of snacking while you watch TV or talk on the phone, or you might overeat before you realize it. Pay attention to what and how much you eat, so your snack is enjoyable and satisfying. And only snack if you're hungry, not just out of habit.

Fats Explained – What To Avoid

What is dietary fat? Fat is an essential part of the human diet, but some forms of it are unhealthy. Here's what you need to know:

Monounsaturated Fat

This type of fat lowers low-density lipoproteins, or bad cholesterol, and raises high-density lipoproteins, or good cholesterol. It is liquid at room temperature and is found in olives, olive oil, canola oil, cashews, almonds, peanuts and most other nuts, and avocados.

Polyunsaturated Fat

Polyunsaturated fat lowers LDL and raises HDL. It is liquid at room temperature and is found in corn, soybean, safflower and cottonseed oils and fish.

Saturated Fat

This type of fat raises both LDL and HDL and is solid at room temperature. It is found in whole milk, butter, cheese, ice cream, meat, chocolate, coconuts, coconut milk and coconut oil.

Trans Fat

The least healthy fat, trans fat raises LDL and is solid or semi-solid at room temperature. It is found in most margarines, vegetable shortening, partially hydrogenated vegetable oil, deep-fried chips, many fast foods and most commercial baked goods.

Hidden Time Bombs – How To Diffuse Them

If you are trying to lose weight, you should limit on fat and sodium intake. You should not eat the following foods.

Red meats, oils (all kinds high in saturated fats, and margarine), salad dressings with oil, full fat dairy products, alcohol, brownies, all type of sugar, and any food with more than 2 gram of fat per serving.

Alcohol increases your weight. A daily dose of 12 oz beer can (146 calories) can increase your weight by 1.2 pounds in just 4 weeks if you don't do any exercise!

Avoid meat as these are loaded with saturated fats. For example, a 3 oz beef contains over 300 calories and 80 mg of cholesterol. Bologna gives calories mostly from fat, as high as 80%.

Keep away from cakes. A 3 oz piece of a pound cake gives you over 360 calories, of which more than 50% comes from fat! Even a fat-free pound cake of the same weight gives you 240 calories! Chocolate cakes are not far behind. Cholesterol in cakes

Do you like chocolate and milk bars? Note that a 1.5 oz Kit Kat bar contains 226 calories, of which 49% comes from fat.

Fast food lovers note: McDonald's Big Mac, 7.6 oz contains 590 calories (52% from fat) and 1090 mg sodium. Chicken breast, 3 oz battered, fried, with skin contains 220 calories (47% from fat).

French fries: A regular serving of French fries gives you 237 calories (46% from fat).

Hot Dogs & Sausage: Hot dogs are as bad as bologna. Most of their calories come from fat, as high as 82%. Vegetarian sausage are far better as they contain much less fat.

Potato Chips: They are the worst as they contain too much fat and too much salt. 10 chips gives you over 100 calories, of which 55 calories come from fat. Instead, try pretzels (remove salt) and air-popped popcorn. Avoid high sodium foods.

Donuts: An average size glazed donut gives you 242 calories; half of this goes to your waistline.

Eggs: One fully boiled, large egg gives you 79 calories and 216 mg cholesterol. Eat eggs in moderation, particularly if you are watching your cholesterol.

Ice Creams: Some of the ice creams are not recommended. For example, 1 scoop of Vanilla ice cream, premium (Baskin-Robbins), gives you 250 calories, of which 150 calories comes from fat. Try the mango ice cream instead.

Nuts: Though a handful of nuts are recommended, too much is not good for weight loss. For example, a handful dried macadamia contains 235 calories, 88% of this comes from fat. Nuts Nutrition

Pies: Some of the pies are loaded with fat. For example, a Pecan pie contains more than 500 calories of which over 45% comes from fat.

The Label is Your New CSI

Tips for Using the Food Label

Most packaged foods have a Nutrition Facts label. Here are some tips for reading the label and making smart food choices:

Check servings and calories. Look at the serving size and how many servings you are actually eating.

Tip: If you eat 2 servings of a food, you will consume double the calories and double the % Daily Value (% DV) of the nutrients listed on the Nutrition Facts Label.

Make your calories count. Look at the calories on the label and compare them with the nutrients they offer.

Tip: When you look at a food's nutrition label, first check the calories, and then check the nutrients to decide whether the food is worth eating.

Eat less sugar. Foods with added sugars may provide calories, but few essential nutrients. So, look for foods and beverages low in added sugars. Read the ingredient list, and make sure added sugars are not one of the first few ingredients.

Tip: Names for added sugars (caloric sweeteners) include sucrose, glucose, high fructose corn syrup, corn syrup, maple syrup, and fructose.

Know your fats. Look for foods low in saturated and *trans* fats, and cholesterol, to help reduce the risk of heart disease. Most of the fats you eat should be polyunsaturated and monounsaturated fats, such as those in fish, nuts, and vegetable oils.

Tip: Fat should be in the range of 20% to 35% of the calories you eat.

Reduce sodium (salt); increase potassium. Research shows that eating less than 2,300 milligrams of sodium (about 1 tsp of salt) per day may reduce the risk of high blood pressure. Older adults tend to be salt-sensitive. If you are older adult or salt-sensitive, aim to eat no more than 1,500 milligrams of sodium each day—the equivalent of about 3/4 teaspoon. To meet the daily potassium recommendation of at least 4,700 milligrams, consume fruits and vegetables, and fat-free and low-fat milk products that are sources of potassium including: sweet potatoes, beet greens, white potatoes, white beans, plain yogurt, prune juice, and bananas. These counteract some of sodium's effects on blood pressure.

Tip: Most sodium you eat is likely to come from processed foods, not from the salt shaker. Read the Nutrition Facts Label, and choose foods lower in sodium and higher in potassium.

Use the % Daily Value (% DV) column: 5% DV or less is low, and 20% DV or more is high.

Keep these low: saturated and trans fats, cholesterol, and sodium.

Get enough of these: potassium and fiber, vitamins A, C, and D, calcium, and iron.

Check the calories: 400 or more calories per serving of a single food item is high.

Nutrition Facts

Serving Size 1 cup (228g)
Servings Per Container 2

Amount Per Serving

Calories 250   Calories from Fat 110

	% Daily Value*
Total Fat 12g	**18%**
Saturated Fat 3g	**15%**
Trans Fat 3g	
Cholesterol 30mg	**10%**
Sodium 470mg	**20%**
Potassium 700mg	**20%**
Total Carbohydrate 31g	**10%**
Dietary Fiber 0g	**0%**
Sugars 5g	
Protein 5g	

Vitamin A	**4%**
Vitamin C	**2%**
Calcium	**20%**
Iron	**4%**

* Percent Daily Values are based on a 2,000 calorie diet. Your Daily Values may be higher or lower depending on your calorie needs.

	Calories:	2,000	2,500
Total Fat	Less than	65g	80g
Sat Fat	Less than	20g	25g
Cholesterol	Less than	300mg	300mg
Sodium	Less than	2,400mg	2,400mg
Total Carbohydrate		300g	375g
Dietary Fiber		25g	30g

Start here

Check calories

Quick guide to % DV

5% or less is low
20% or more is high

Limit these

Get enough of these

Footnote

Customizing Your Meal Plan

Because diet goals are different for each person, only you can customize a meal plan that is right for you. A wonderful free online tool to use to accomplish this is located at the U.S. Department of Agriculture's website.

http://www.mypyramid.gov/mypyramid/index.aspx

Plan Your Day the Easy Way

It is essential to the success of your weight control program to Think Ahead and apply The FTP Principle: "Fail To Plan Means Plan To Fail."

One of the best ways to have a healthy diet is to prepare your own food and eat in regularly. Pick a few healthy recipes that you and your family like and build a meal schedule around them. If you have three or four meals planned per week and eat leftovers on the other nights, you will be much farther ahead than if you are eating out or having frozen dinners most nights.

In general, healthy eating ingredients are found around the outer edges of most grocery stores—fresh fruits and vegetables, fish and poultry, whole grain breads and dairy products. The centers of many grocery stores are filled with overpriced, processed foods that aren't good for you. Shop the perimeter of the store for most of your groceries (fresh items), add a few things from the freezer section (frozen fruits and vegetables), and the aisles with spices, oils, and whole grains (like rolled oats, brown rice, whole wheat pasta).

Try to cook one or both weekend days or on a weekday evening and make extra to freeze or set aside for another night. Cooking ahead saves time and money, and it is gratifying to know that you have a home cooked meal waiting to be eaten.

Challenge yourself to come up with two or three dinners that can be put together without going to the store—utilizing things in your pantry, freezer and spice rack. A delicious dinner of whole grain pasta with a quick tomato sauce or a quick and easy black bean quesadilla on a whole wheat flour tortilla (among endless other recipes) could act as your go-to meal when you are just too busy to shop or cook.

Stock your kitchen to be meal ready!

Try to keep your kitchen stocked with recipe basics:

Fresh and frozen fruits and vegetables.

Recipe and soup starters such as garlic, onions, carrots, and celery.

Healthy staples like brown rice, white Basmati rice, whole-wheat pasta, quinoa, and wild rice.

Whole wheat bread and tortillas for healthy sandwiches and wraps.

Beans such as lentils, black beans, chickpeas, black-eyed peas, kidney beans, fava beans, and lima beans.

Frozen corn, peas, and other vegetables to add to recipes or for a quick vegetable side dish.

Frozen fruit and berries to make smoothies or frozen desserts.

Dark greens for salads, plus salad add-ins like dried fruit, nuts, beans, and seeds.

Fresh and dried herbs and spices.

Healthy fats and oils for cooking, such as olive oil and canola oil. You can also try specialty oils like peanut, sesame, or truffle oil for adding flavor.

Unsalted nuts for snacking, like almonds, walnuts, cashews, peanuts, and pistachios.

Vinegars, such as balsamic, red wine, and rice vinegar for salads and veggies.

Strong cheeses, like aged Parmesan or blue cheese for intense flavor in salads, pasta, and soups.

Plan your meals and snacks a week in advance and shop accordingly. Taking an hour or two per week to plan, shop and prepare your meal plan is well worth the time. This allows you to anticipate problem times in your day for eating and plan for them.

Once you do this a few times, it's easy to simply repeat the process by picking up the things you need from the store when you shop.

List the foods you like from each food group, and plan your meals and snacks, keeping in mind the caloric count for each item.

An easy way to save time and money when you cook is to freeze portions of your meals in small Ziploc freezer bags, Ziploc plastic containers or similar storage methods so that meals can be as easy as boiling some water or using the microwave.

There are some excellent "Seal-A-Meal" type appliances on the market that keep food fresher longer in the freezer and allow you to carry them with you in your insulated freezer bag.

Small portion controlled size cans of vegetables are also a good idea for people on the go with limited time.

Smoothies –
Blending Your Way To Fitness

Smoothies can be great for weight loss and make a wonderful breakfast, snack, or meal replacement, provided you are making it yourself. Commercially bought smoothies are often packed with sugar.

Make your own smoothies by taking a blender, adding a banana and other fresh fruits, some ice and some low fat milk You can also add protein powder if you'd like, but limit the milk portion to one cup.

I add wheat germ to mine.

Recipes That Work

Your favorite foods can be prepared in many low-cal and delicious ways if you are so inclined to use recipes for preparing your own meals.

The key is to find recipes that work for you, with foods that you like and that you can prepare efficiently to your unique schedule.

The Food Network offers a great website for healthy eating that is packed with delicious low fat recipes. It can be found at:

http://www.foodnetwork.com/healthy-eating/index.html
Another fantastic recipe site is at:

http://www.lowfatlifestyle.com/entrees/entreeindex.htm

Here is an example:

Apricot Honey Grilled Chicken

Try low fat grilled chicken recipe for a fruity change of pace!
Servings: 4
- 1/3 cup Grey Poupon Honey Mustard
- 3 tablespoons apricot preserves
- 1 teaspoon ground ginger
- 4 skinless, boneless chicken breasts

Blend mustard, preserves and ginger. Brush mixture on chicken. Grill or broil 6 to 8 minutes on each side or until done. Brush frequently with preserve mixture.

Per Serving: 187 Calories
3g Fat (15.0% calories from fat)
29g Protein
11g Carbohydrate
trace Dietary Fiber
68mg Cholesterol
355mg Sodium
Low Fat Recipes Furnished by LowFatLifestyle.com
© - Copyright 2006

EXERCISE –
PROVEN METHOD THAT WORK

The benefits of exercise are well-known, and essential to your weight control program. Not only does exercise make you feel better and live longer, it also helps your mental states. Proper exercise aids in sleep, digestion and has many other benefits.

Recommended Exercise Methods:

A few simple rules are helpful as you develop your own routine.

- Don't eat for 2 hours before vigorous exercise.
- Drink plenty of fluids before, during, and after a workout.
- Adjust your activity level according to the weather, and reduce it when you are fatigued or ill.
- When exercising, listen to the body's warning symptoms, and consult a doctor if exercise causes chest pain, irregular heartbeat, unusual fatigue, nausea, unexpected breathlessness, or light-headedness.

Heart Rate Goal

Heart rate is the standard guide for determining aerobic exercise intensity. It is useful for people training at aerobic intensity, or people with certain cardiac risk factors who have been set a maximum heart rate by their doctor.

You can determine your heart rate by counting your pulse, or by using a heart rate monitor. To feel your own pulse, press the first two fingers of one hand gently down on the inside of the wrist or under the jaw on the right or left side of the front of the neck. You should feel a faint pounding as blood passes through the artery. Each pounding is a beat.

• Resting heart rate: The average heart rate for a person at rest is 60 - 80 beats per minute. It is usually lower for people who are physically fit, and often rises as you get older. You can determine your resting heart rate by counting how many times your heart beats in one minute. The best time to do this is in the morning after a good night's sleep before you get out of bed.

• Maximum heart rate. To determine your own maximum heart rate per minute subtract your age from 220. For example, if you are 45, you would calculate your maximum heart rate as follows: 220 - 45= 175.

• Target heart rate. Your target rate is 50 - 75% of your maximum heart rate. You should measure your pulse off and on while you exercise to make sure you stay within this range. After about 6 months of regular exercise, you may be able to increase your target heart rate to 85% (but only if you can comfortably do so).

Certain heart medications may lower your maximum and target heart rates. Always check with your doctor before starting an exercise program.

Note: Swimmers should use a heart rate target of 75% of the maximum and then subtract 12 beats per minute. The reason for this is that swimming will not raise the heart rate quite as much as other sports because of the so-called "diving reflex," which causes the heart to slow down automatically when the body is immersed in water.

VO2 Max. Serious exercisers may use a VO2 max calculation, which measures the amount of oxygen consumed during intensive, all-out exercise. The most accurate testing method uses computers, but anyone can estimate V02 without instrumentation (with an accuracy of about 95%):

After running at top pace for 15 minutes, round off the distance run to the nearest 25 meters.

Divide that number by 15.

Subtract 133.

Multiply the total by 0.172, then add 33.3.

Olympic and professional athletes train for VO2 max levels above 80. A VO2 max equaling between 50 and 80 is considered an excellent score for overall fitness. For the average person exercising for fitness and health, this value is not necessary.

Warm-Up and Cool-Down

Warming up and cooling down are important parts of every exercise routine. They help the body make the transition from rest to activity and back again, and can help prevent soreness or injury, especially in older people.

Practice warm-up exercises for 5 - 10 minutes at the beginning of an exercise session. Older people need a longer period to warm up their muscles. Strengthening exercises, quiet calisthenics, and walking are ideal.

To cool down, you should walk slowly until the heart rate is 10 - 15 beats above your resting heart rate. Stopping too suddenly can sharply reduce blood pressure, and is dangerous for older people. It may also cause muscle cramping.

Stretching may be appropriate for the cooling down period, but it must be done carefully for warming up because it can injure cold muscles. (There is no clear evidence, however, that stretching reduces muscle injuries.)

Warming up before exercise and cooling down after is just as important as the exercise itself. By properly warming up the muscles and joints with low-level aerobic movement for 5 - 10 minutes one may avoid injury. Cooling down after exercise by walking slowly, then stretching muscles, may also prevent strains and blood pressure fluctuation.

For most people, exercise may be divided into three general categories:
- **Aerobic or endurance**
- **Strength or resistance**
- **Flexibility**

A balanced program should include all three. Speed training is also a major category, but generally only competitive athletes practice it.

Aerobic (Endurance) Training

Benefits of Aerobic Exercise. Regular aerobic exercise provides the following benefits:

• Protection from heart attack, stroke, diabetes, dementia, depression, colon and breast cancers, and early death.

• Builds endurance

• Keeps the heart pumping at a steady and high rate for a long time.

• Boosts HDL ("good") cholesterol levels.

• Helps control blood pressure

• Strengthens the bones in the spine

• Helps maintain normal weight

• Improves one's sense of well-being

Types of Aerobic Exercise:

Aerobic exercise is usually categorized as high or low intensity. High intensity aerobic exercise is further classified as high or low impact. Examples of each include the following:

• Low- to moderate-impact exercises: Walking, swimming, stair climbing, step classes, rowing, and cross-country skiing. Nearly anyone in reasonable health can engage in some low- to moderate-impact exercise. Brisk walking burns as many calories as jogging for the same distance and poses less risk for injury to muscle and bone.

• High-impact exercises: Running, dance exercise, tennis, racquetball, squash. Perform high-impact exercises no more often than every other day, and less often for those who are overweight, elderly, out of condition, or have an injury or other medical problem that would rule out high-impact.

4 hours per week are best. Some research indicates that simply walking briskly for 3 or more hours a week reduces the risk for coronary heart disease by 45%. In general, the following guidelines are useful for most individuals:

For most healthy young adults, the best approach is a mix of low- and higher-impact exercise. Two weekly workouts will maintain fitness, but three to five sessions a week are better.

People who are out of shape or elderly should start aerobic training gradually. For example, they may start with 5 - 10 minutes of low-impact aerobic activity every other day and build toward a goal of 30 minutes per day, three to seven times a week. (For heart protection, weekly total is the key.)

Swimming is an ideal exercise for many elderly people, and for certain people with physical limitations. People with physical limitations include pregnant women, individuals with muscle, joint, or bone problems, and those who suffer from exercise-induced asthma.

People who seek to lose weight should concentrate on calories burnt each week, not the number of workout sessions.

One way of gauging the aerobic intensity of exercise is to aim for a "talking pace," which is enough to work up a sweat and still be able to converse with a friend without gasping for breath. As fitness increases, the "talking pace" will become faster and faster.

All that's really necessary for a workout is a good pair of shoes that are made well and fit well. They should be broken in, but not worn down. They should support the ankle and provide cushioning for walking as well as for impact sports such as running or aerobic dancing.

Airing out the shoes and feet after exercising reduces chances for skin conditions such as athlete's foot.

Clothing: Comfort and safety are the key words for workout clothing. For outdoor nighttime exercise, a reflective vest and light-colored clothing must be worn. Bikers, inline skaters, and equestrians should always wear safety devices such as helmets, wrist guards, and knee and elbow pads.

Goggles are mandatory for indoor racquet sports. For vigorous athletic activities, such as football, ankle braces may be more effective than tape in preventing ankle injuries.

Aerobic-Exercise Equipment: Home aerobic exercise machines can be adapted to any fitness level and used day or night. Before investing in any exercise machine, however, it is wise to first test it at a gym. In addition, initial supervised training when using these machines can reduce the risk of injury that might occur with self-instruction.

Very inexpensive exercise machines tend to be flimsy and hard to adjust, but many sturdy machines are available at moderate prices. The higher-end models may utilize computers to record calories burned, speed, and mileage. Their readouts may provide motivation and gauge the intensity of a workout, however, they are not always accurate.

The following are a few observations on specific equipment:

• A good floor mat is important to provide cushioning for all home exercises.

• A simple jump rope improves aerobic endurance for people who are able to perform high-impact exercise. Jumping rope should be done on a floor mat plus a surface that has some give to avoid joint injury.

• For burning calories, the treadmill has been ranked best, followed by stair climbers, the rowing machine, cross-country ski machine, and stationary bicycle. (Elliptical trainers, however, may be even better than treadmills for increasing heart rate, calorie expenditure, and oxygen consumption.)

• Stationary bikes condition leg muscles and are fairly economical and easy to use safely. The pedals should turn smoothly, the seat height should adjust easily, and the bike's computer should be able to adjust intensity.

• Stair machines also condition leg muscles. They offer very intense, low-impact workouts and may be as effective as running with less chance of injury.

• Rowing and cross-country ski machines exercise both the upper and lower body.

Strength or Resistance Training

Benefits of Strength Exercise

While aerobic exercise increases endurance and helps the heart, it does not build upper body strength or tone muscles. Strength-training exercises provide the following benefits:
- Build muscle strength while burning fat
- Help maintain bone density
- It is also associated with a lower risk for heart disease, possibly because it lowers LDL (the so-called "bad" cholesterol) levels.

Strength exercise is beneficial for everyone, even people in there 90s. It is the only form of exercise that can slow and even reverse the decline in muscle mass, bone density, and strength that occur with aging.

Please note: People at risk for cardiovascular disease should not perform strength exercises without checking with a doctor.

Types of Muscle Contractions

There are three types of muscle contractions involved in strength training:
- Isometric contractions do not change the length of the muscle. An example is pushing against a wall.
- Concentric contractions shorten muscles. An example is the "up" phase of the biceps curl.
- Eccentric contractions lengthen muscles. An example is the "down" phase as weights are lowered.

Strength-Training Regimens

Strength training involves intense and short-duration activities. For beginners, adding 10 - 20 minutes of modest strength training two to three times a week may be appropriate. The following are some guidelines for starting a strength regimen:

The sequence of a strength training session should begin with training large muscles and multiple joints at higher intensity, and end with small muscle and single joint exercises at lower intensities.

You should perform both shortening and lengthening muscle actions. Emphasizing the movements that lengthen muscles is of increasing interest. This approach involves slowing and increasing the duration of these "down" movements. It appears to significantly increase blood flow, and some evidence suggests it may achieve stronger muscles more quickly.

It may also improve heart function compared to standard movements. Exercises that lengthen muscles may be particularly beneficial for older people and some people with chronic health problems.

This type of training increases the risk for muscle soreness and injury, however, and this approach is still controversial.

Strength training involves moving specific muscles in the same pattern against a resisting force (such as a weight) for a preset number of times.

This is called a repetition. People should first choose a weight that is about half of what would require a maximum effort in one repetition. In other words, if it would take maximum effort to do a single repetition with a 10-pound dumbbell, the person would start with a five-pound dumbbell. In the beginning, most people can start with one set of 8 - 15 repetitions per muscle group with low weights. As individuals are able to perform one or two repetitions over their routine, weights can be increased by 2 - 10%.

Breathe slowly and rhythmically. Exhale as the movement begins. Inhale when returning to the starting point.

The first half of each repetition typically lasts 2 - 3 seconds. The return to the original position lasts 4 seconds.

Joints should be moved rhythmically through their full range of motion during a repetition. Do not lock up the joint while exercising it.

For maximum benefit, one should allow 48 hours between workouts for full muscle recovery.

Strength-Training Equipment

Unlike aerobic exercise, strength training almost always requires some equipment. Strength-training equipment does not, however, have to cost anything.

Any heavy object that can be held in the hand, such as a plastic bottle filled with sand or water, can serve as a weight.

Dumbbells (1 - 10 pounds) and resistance bands are inexpensive, portable, and effective.

Wearable weights help strengthen and tone the upper body.

Ankle weights strengthen and tone muscles in the lower body. They should not be worn during high-impact aerobics or jumping.

Hand grips strengthen arms and are good for relieving tension.

A pull-up bar can be mounted in a doorway for chin-ups and pull-ups.

More elaborate and expensive home equipment for working body muscles is also available, costing from $100 to over $1,000. No one should purchase or use strength-training equipment without instruction from a professional.

Flexibility Training (Stretching)

Benefits of Flexibility Training

Flexibility training uses stretching exercises. Many stretching exercises are particularly beneficial for the back. In general, flexibility training provides the following benefits:

• Prevents cramps, stiffness, and injuries

• Improves joint and muscle movement (improved range of motion)

Certain flexibility practices, such as yoga and tai chi, also involve meditation and breathing techniques that reduce stress. Such practices appear to have many health and mental benefits.

They may be very suitable and highly beneficial for older people, and for patients with certain chronic diseases.

Flexibility Training Regimens

Doctors recommend performing stretching exercises for 10 - 12 minutes at least three times a week. The following are some general guidelines:
- When stretching, exhale and extend the muscles to the point of tension, not pain, and hold for 20 - 60 seconds. (Beginners may need to start with a 5- to 10-second stretch.)
- Breathe evenly and constantly while holding the stretch.
- Inhale when returning to a relaxed position. Holding your breath defeats the purpose; it causes muscle contraction and raises blood pressure.
- When doing stretches that involve the back, relax the spine to keep the lower back flush with the mat, and to work only the muscles required for changing position (often these are only the abdominal muscles).

Specific Exercise Tips for Older People

Studies continue to show that it is never too late to start exercising. Elderly adults who exercise twice a week can significantly increased their body strength, flexibility, balance, and agility. Studies show that even small improvements in physical fitness and activity can prolong life and independent living.

A recent study based on a 35-year follow-up showed that in men who increased their physical activity at age 50, the reduction in mortality rate was similar to that of smoking cessation. In fact, after 10 years of increased physical activity, these men had the same mortality rate for their age group as men who were highly physically active throughout entire adult their lives.

Still, about half of Americans over 60 describe themselves as sedentary (inactive). According to a 2004 report by the Centers for Disease Control and Prevention, about 12% of people aged 65 - 75 years, and 10% of people aged 75 years or older, meet current recommendations for strength training.

The following tips for exercising may be helpful:

Any older person should have a complete physical and medical examination, as well as professional instruction, before starting an exercise program.

Start low and go slow. For sedentary, older people, one or more of the following programs may be helpful and safe: Low-impact aerobics, gait (step) training, balance exercises, tai chi, self-paced walking, and lower legs resistance training, using elastic tubing or ankle weights.

Even in the nursing home, programs aimed at improving strength, balance, gait, and flexibility have significant benefits.

Strength training assumes even more importance as one ages, because after age 30 everyone undergoes a slow process of muscular weakening (atrophy).

This process can be reduced or even reversed by adding resistance training to an exercise program. As little as 1 day a week of resistance training improves overall strength and agility. Strength training also improves heart and blood vessel health.

Flexibility exercises promote healthy muscle growth and help reduce the stiffness and loss of balance that accompanies aging.

Chair exercises may be performed by people who are unable to walk.

Older women are at risk for incontinence accidents during exercise. This can be reduced or prevented by performing Kegel exercises, limiting fluids (without risking dehydration), going to the bathroom frequently, and using leakage prevention pads or insertable devices.

Jane Fonda Workout and At Home Videos

Whatever your opinion of Jane Fonda, she was the first woman to capitalize on the home workout video, and revolutionized an industry. Buying one of her workout videos is an excellent investment. Not only does it allow you to save time and money working out at home, it also gets you started on following a working routine without being self-conscious.

All you need is a good pair of workout shoes, A DVD player, TV and a towel and you're off to the races!

Her routines are remarkably effective, and for me and my husband it got us working out when we never thought we would.

Whether you are doing it with a partner or on your own, workout videos are a great way to go. Experiment with different ones until you find one that works for you.

The only drawback I see in using workout videos is that it's easy to get lazy and not follow the regimen as directed, or worse yet, skip working out altogether.

This is why many people choose to go to a gym and utilize the services at the gym of a workout trainer, to insure you have a commitment you need to show up for, and someone there to push you when you will inevitably want to fall short of finishing your routine.

Gyms and Why They Are The Best Investment You Can Make In Your Health

With the proliferation of nationwide chains such as "24 Hour Fitness" and "Ballys Total Fitness," it puts location and convenience in your court and makes working out an affordable and fun routine.

For prices as low as $20 a month you can avail yourself of great workout equipment, classes, and even a pool, sauna and whirlpool at some locations.

It also can be temptation to socialize, and while chatting with a nearby patron can help the workout time go faster, it can easily become a habit that can detract from the effectiveness of your workout.

I make it a point to be courteous and respectful of people, but I avoid making social contacts there, which is just a personal preference for me. I found when I used to be conversational with people I was working out near, it made me feel obligated to socialize with these same people each time I'd see them on future visits.

You be surprised at how quickly this can turn into "Hi hello how are you" with far more people than you'd ever realized, and then becomes a burden that can distract you from your routine.

People will burn up your time in a heartbeat and think nothing of it, but isn't time the most precious commodity we have?

Personal trainers are an option for those who find their own self-discipline lacking, and need to take a large amount of weight off quickly.

Beware, though that the real bread and butter for the gym chains are selling you personal training services, and some of the locations can be pretty aggressive in getting you to buy their often over-priced plans.

You can avail yourself of the "free workout consultation" with a personal trainer to learn the methods used to set up your routine, but be prepared for the sales pitch that will inevitably come afterwards.

Who knows, you might find a personal training program well worth your money if you absolutely need someone to "light a fire under your bottom" and cannot seem to get results on your own.

Fitness Trainers: Luxury or Necessity?

The U.S. Department of Labor estimates that in 2006 there were nearly 250,000 personal fitness trainers employed in the U.S. In the next ten years, that's expected to grow nearly 25 percent.

Yet despite their growing popularity, hiring a personal fitness trainer isn't for everyone.

Although some gyms and health clubs provide free personal fitness training services, most personal trainers come with a price tag. Depending on your location, that could run you anywhere from $30 - $70 a session — and sometimes even more in certain fitness clubs and locations.

So is it worth it?

Is a trainer really necessary?
The answer is that "it depends."

Personal Trainers: Great for Beginners

If you are just starting a workout routine, a couple of sessions with a personal trainer can reap big rewards over the long haul.

A good trainer will spend time with you taking a close look at your current fitness levels and will perform a thorough evaluation of your diet, nutrition and activity levels. They will also look at any pre-existing medical conditions and injuries, and your personal fitness goals. From all of this information, they'll create a custom workout and diet plan that will help you achieve those goals.

Even more important, hitting the gym for the first time can be an intimidating experience.

An effective personal trainer will also spend time familiarizing you with the equipment in the gym and matching you up with the right exercises for your experience level and fitness goals. They can also help demonstrate the right form to use when performing exercises, which will increase your chances of success, while reducing your chance of injury.

But I Already Know What to Do In The Gym. How Can A Personal Trainer Help Me?

Even if you have plenty of experience in the gym, a personal trainer can still come in handy — especially when you find your progress stalling. Even the most seasoned fitness buffs can get in a rut, and sometimes having a pair of fresh eyes on your workout regimen can be the difference between a short-term setback and a more lengthy plateau.

There are trainers that specialize in certain areas, such as strength or weight training, rehabilitation, sports- or recreation-specific training, or bodybuilding, who can provide valuable outside perspective and expertise. Sometimes all it takes to jump-start a stale workout routine is a little kick in the ass. Having that voice over your shoulder is often all it takes.

Personal Fitness Training for Special Needs

The personal training field is no longer just populated by generalists. There are a number of highly-qualified, highly-trained professionals who specialize in fields like rehabilitative exercise, sports training and conditioning and even fitness training for the obese.

For example, if you are looking to bring your golf game up, there are sports conditioning trainers who can develop personalized training plans to improve your swing, strength and performance when you are on the green.

If you are recovering from an injury, there are trainers who specialize in rehabilitative training and can help you regain strength and mobility. If you are struggling with your weight, there are trainers who do nothing but work with overweight individuals to help them gradually (and sanely) reduce body fat.

The key here is to find a personal trainer that meets your individual needs.

Do I Have to Have A Personal Trainer to Be Successful?

Having a personal trainer will not guarantee success. They can only create a roadmap for you and help you stay focused on your goals. The rest is really up to you.

Depending on your motivation levels, knowledge and desire to learn more about fitness, you may never need to use a personal trainer. There are plenty of highly-fit people who never employ personal trainers and achieve very impressive results. On the other hand, there are individuals who use trainers regularly who still find themselves slacking off at home on their diet, and are disappointed with their results.

At the end of the day, it really comes down to the effort and dedication that you put in, regardless of who is training you.

Some people are highly self-motivated, while others need a little day-to-day, guidance. If you fall into the self-motivated camp, you'll likely find that using a personal trainer only gives you marginal gains over your usual workout regimen. On the other hand, if you are finding it difficult to keep your focus up and stay positive, a personal trainer can be just the ticket.

Toys and Traps – Gadgets and Gadflies

Since time began, it seems like there has been someone hawking the latest exercise device. There were probably early caveman version of "abdo-rollers" and "thigh-masters" made with Flintstones-type ingenuity, but in the end, it's all about getting your money and leaving you flabby and broke.

Marketers know that you are more apt to buy such gadgets because in your mind you think you are going to use them, and you believe they are going to work.

Most of all they are trying to sell you the notion of easy results.

It will probably come as little surprise to you that much of the time these devices end up sitting in a closet.

The gadflies are everywhere, people who are self-proclaimed experts (or former athletes or movie stars) on fitness and hawking the latest program, device, book, diet or fad gadget.

My advice is to avoid these tempting distractions and stick to the basic methods that are proven to work. There is nothing these gadgets offer that can't be accomplished just as easily if not more effectively simply doing the basic version of the same exercise.

SIDEBAR: Do Ab Machines Shown on TV Really Work? – A Report from ABC News.com

Do those gadgets really give you flat abs or a six-pack stomach?

When commercials for those gadgets that claim to trim and strengthen the abdomen come on, out-of-shape viewers can't help but feel a jolt of guilt about their expanding waistline and, perhaps, their long-running absence from the gym. But then comes the sweet promise that they can slim down, without breaking a sweat.

"Just 10 minutes with Fast-Abs is equivalent of up to 600 sit-ups," the commercial announcer says, as images of buff bodies are shown on screen. "Now you can work out your abs anywhere — watching TV, at the office, even around the house."

From coast to coast, the airwaves are bloated with gadgets like the "Ab-Energizer," "Fast Abs" and "The AbTronic" that promise to shape up your abdominal muscles, even without exercise. The marketers claim that ab gadget devotees will find themselves with bodies like Superman or Wonder Woman, but critics say it isn't so.

Good Morning America 's consumer correspondent Greg Hunter found that the machines can cause minor skin burns. Experts told him that anyone who thinks that the devices alone will turn them into Mr. Universe is mistaken. The gadgets are based on electronic muscle stimulation, or EMS, a system that delivers an electric charge to make muscles contract.

John Porcari, a professor of exercise and sports science at the University of Wisconsin, tested an EMS device similar to those on the market in a study commissioned by the American Council on Exercise. After eight weeks of using the device only, participants had no significant increases in muscle size or strength.

"I think people are wasting their time," Porcari said. "I think they're better off spending their money on a personal trainer or buying a membership to a health club, or buying a home piece of exercise equipment that they're going to use."

AbTronic declined any comment under advice of their attorney. Ab-Energizer also declined comment, and Fast-Abs did not return phone calls or e-mails sent by Good Morning America .

Want Flat Abs? Order Now

The Fast-Abs ad claims the technology makes it easy: "It's like our engineer shrunk half a gym of bulky, expensive exercise equipment into a little electronic miracle the size of a pack of matches."

Victoria Delaney, a San Francisco Bay area woman who saw the AbTronic infomercial, was intrigued by the thought of achieving amazing abs just like the young woman in the commercial.

"That's what I thought I was going to get," Delaney told Hunter, pointing to the buff young woman's flat stomach. After seeing the ad, she immediately reached for her telephone and credit card and ordered an AbTronic.

Delaney thought the device would let her get trim while sitting around and reading a book or watching TV.

"Sure, I thought it would be easy," Delaney said.

Company Warns of Skin Burning Reports

Delaney said she used her AbTronic religiously for three days, but then she said she had to stop because it gave her a number of minor but painful burns on her arms, stomach, both legs and her back, making it difficult to sit.

When she looked at the instruction booklet later, Delaney discovered that the company warned that "skin irritation and burns ... have been reported."

Though Delaney does not have any permanent injuries, her pride is a little scarred, and she feels naïve for being taken, she said.

But it is easy to see why people like Delaney might be drawn to the devices. Not only does the AbTronic infomercial show seemingly perfect men and women using it, the commercials claim that a University of Maryland study backs up products like theirs.

"Their conclusion was that an electronic stimulation was much better than exercise alone, whether you use it as a supplement to your normal workout, or just by itself," a female co-host of the infomercial says. "That proves that you get better results by the use of the AbTronic fitness system," the male co-host chimes in.

Machine Can't Do It Alone

The University of Maryland scientist who conducted the study, Dr. Gad Alon, published an article about electronic muscle stimulation in 1987. He said that he believes high-quality EMS devices can strengthen the abdominal muscles, but that the AbTronic infomercial took his findings out of context.

"In fact, we have used electrical stimulation on abdominal strengthening in a number of studies," he said. "And that particular one [AbTronic] does not look at all like the type of strengthening we do with electrical stimulation."

Porcari acknowledges that medically approved EMS devices can play a useful role in rehabilitative medicine. But he says consumers can't comfortably get strong enough contractions from these infomercial devices to build "awesome abs" without real exercise.

"To get the benefits, you have to make your muscles contract to a certain level, and that requires you to be able to withstand a lot of pain," he said.

Dr. Julio Garcia, a Las Vegas plastic surgeon, appeared in the AbTronic infomercial touting the device.

"The nice thing about the AbTronic system is you don't have to go to a gymnasium, where you have to do weight-lifting exercises, where we may have some other medical problems that prevent from doing that — whether it's high blood pressure or bad joints," Garcia says in the infomercial.

Garcia told Hunter that although EMS. can help maintain muscle tone, it will not help people lose weight. He also said that the AbTronic commercial took some of his words out of context, and that the machine alone cannot help a person lose weight, lose inches and gain muscle definition.

"It was my intent to talk about many things together — diet, exercise, and the machine," Garcia said. "It has apparently been portrayed as just a machine itself. And that's not what I was there to talk about."

Delaney says she spent $150 on the AbTronic, and chalks it up to one of life's lessons that she hopes others can learn from. Her advice to anyone lured by the ab machine commercials is simple

"Don't buy it," she said.

SIDEBAR: A Guide to Personal Change – US Department of Health and Human Services

Your Weight Is Important

Over the past few years it has become clear that weight is an important health issue. Some people who need to lose weight

91

for their health don't recognize it, while others who don't need to lose weight want to get thinner for cosmetic reasons. We understand that in some ways your weight is different from, for example, your cholesterol level or your blood pressure, because you can't see what these are by looking at someone. Many patients have had health care providers who approached their weight in a less-than-sensitive or helpful manner. Some patients may have had health care encounters in which they felt blamed, but not helped. Successful weight management is a long-term challenge.

Weight can affect a person's self-esteem. Excess weight is highly visible and evokes some powerful reactions, however unfairly, from other people and from the people who carry the excess weight. The amount of weight loss needed to improve your health may be much less than you wish to lose, when you consider how you evaluate your weight. Research has shown that your health can be greatly improved by a loss of 5–10 percent of your starting weight. That doesn't mean you have to stop there, but it does mean that an initial goal of losing 5–10 percent of your starting weight is both realistic and valuable.

Behaviors That Will Help You Lose Weight and Maintain It

Set the Right Goals.

Setting the right goals is an important first step. Most people trying to lose weight focus on just that one goal: weight loss. However, the most productive areas to focus on are the dietary and physical activity changes that will lead to long-term weight change. Successful weight managers are those who select two or three goals at a time that are manageable.

Useful goals should be (1) specific; (2) attainable (doable); and (3) forgiving (less than perfect). "Exercise more" is a great goal, but it's not specific. "Walk 5 miles every day" is specific and measurable, but is it doable if you're just starting out? "Walk 30 minutes every day" is more attainable, but what happens if you're held up at work one day and there's a thunderstorm during your walking time another day? "Walk 30 minutes, 5 days each week" is specific, doable, and forgiving. In short, a great goal!

Nothing Succeeds Like Success

Shaping is a behavioral technique in which you select a series of short-term goals that get closer and closer to the ultimate goal (e.g., an initial reduction of fat intake from 40 percent of calories to 35 percent of calories, and later to 30 percent). It is based on the concept that "nothing succeeds like success." Shaping uses two important behavioral principles: (1) consecutive goals that move you ahead in small steps are the best way to reach a distant point; and (2) consecutive rewards keep the overall effort invigorated.

Reward Success (But Not With Food)

An effective reward is something that is desirable, timely, and dependent on meeting your goal. The rewards you choose may be material (e.g., a movie or music CD, or a payment toward buying a more costly item) or an act of self-kindness (e.g., an afternoon off from work or just an hour of quiet time away from family). Frequent small rewards, earned for meeting smaller goals, are more effective than bigger rewards that require a long, difficult effort.

Balance Your Food Checkbook

"Self-monitoring" refers to observing and recording some aspect of your behavior, such as calorie intake, servings of fruits and vegetables, amount of physical activity, etc., or an outcome of these behaviors, such as weight. Self-monitoring of a behavior can be used at times when you're not sure how you're doing, and at times when you want the behavior to improve. Self-monitoring of a behavior usually moves you closer to the desired direction and can produce "real-time" records for review by you and your health care provider. For example, keeping a record of your physical activity can let you and your provider know quickly how you're doing. When the record shows that your activity is increasing, you'll be encouraged to keep it up. Some patients find that specific self-monitoring forms make it easier, while others prefer to use their own recording system.

While you may or may not wish to weigh yourself frequently while losing weight, regular monitoring of your weight will be essential to help you maintain your lower weight. When keeping a record of your weight, a graph may be more informative than a list of your weights. When weighing yourself and keeping a weight graph or table, however, remember that one day's diet and exercise patterns won't have a measurable effect on your weight the next day. Today's weight is not a true measure of how well you followed your program yesterday, because your body's water weight will change from day to day, and water changes are often the result of things that have nothing to do with your weight-management efforts.

Avoid a Chain Reaction

Stimulus (cue) control involves learning what social or environmental cues seem to encourage undesired eating, and then changing those cues. For example, you may learn from reflection or from self-monitoring records that you're more likely to overeat while watching television, or whenever treats are on display by the office coffee pot, or when around a certain friend. You might then try to change the situation, such as by separating the association of eating from the cue (don't eat while watching television), avoiding or eliminating the cue (leave the coffee room immediately after pouring coffee), or changing the circumstances surrounding the cue (plan to meet your friend in a nonfood setting). In general, visible and reachable food items are often cues for unplanned eating.

Get the Fullness Message

Changing the way you go about eating can make it easier to eat less without feeling deprived. It takes 15 or more minutes for your brain to get the message that you've been fed. Eating slowly will help you feel satisfied. Eating lots of vegetables and fruits can make you feel fuller. Another trick is to use smaller plates so that moderate portions do not appear too small. Changing your eating schedule, or setting one, can be helpful, especially if you tend to skip, or delay, meals and overeat later.

Conclusion

I've kept this book concise and easy to read and understand so that you may easily absorb what you have read and can begin to apply it right away.

It will also serve as a handy reference book, ideal for keeping a copy in the glove compartment of your vehicle, so that when you are out and about you can refresh your memory and to refer to the calorie and nutrition charts for all the major fast food restaurants.

You are now armed with everything you need to know to start losing weight and keeping it off; all the tricks and tips you need to Staying Thin In A Fast Food World!

Good luck and much success in your journey toward better health, fitness and happiness!

APPENDIX:

Fast Food Nutrition Information:
Charts and Tables From Each Fast Food Restaurant

FAST FOOD RESTAURANTS
NUTRITION CHARTS:

Arby's Menu	Total Calories	Fat Calories	Total Fat (g)	Sat. Fat (g)	Chol. (mg)	Sodium (mg)	Carbs (g)	Protein (g)
Arby's Melt w/Cheddar	340	139	15	5	70	890	36	16
Arby's Arby-Q	360	130	14	4	70	1530	40	16
Arby's Beef 'N Cheddar	480	221	24	8	90	1240	43	23
Arby's Big Montana	630	290	32	15	155	2080	41	47
Arby's Giant Roast Beef	480	206	23	10	110	1440	41	32
Arby's Junior Roast Beef	310	121	13	4.5	70	740	34	16
Arby's Regular Roast Beef	350	151	16	6	85	950	34	21
Arby's Super Roast Beef	470	207	23	7	85	1130	47	22
Arby's Chicken Bacon 'N Swiss	610	293	33	8	110	1550	49	31
Arby's Chicken Breast Fillet	540	265	30	5	90	1160	47	24
Arby's Chicken Cordon Bleu	630	309	35	8	120	1820	47	34
Arby's Grilled Chicken Deluxe	450	198	22	4	110	1050	37	29
Arby's Roast Chicken Club	520	260	28	7	115	1440	38	29
Arby's Hot Ham 'N Swiss	340	119	13	4.5	90	1450	35	23
Arby's French Dip	440	158	18	8	100	1680	42	28
Arby's Hot Ham 'N Swiss	530	239	27	8	110	1860	45	29
Arby's Italian	780	468	53	15	120	2440	49	29
Arby's Philly Beef 'N Swiss	700	378	42	15	130	1940	46	36
Arby's Roast Beef	760	426	48	16	130	2230	47	35
Arby's Turkey	630	328	37	9	100	2170	51	26
Arby's Roast Beef & Swiss	810	381	42	13	130	1780	73	37
Arby's Roast Ham & Swiss	730	307	34	8	125	2180	74	36

Arby's Roast Chicken Caesar	820	336	38	9	140	2160	75	43
Arby's Roast Turkey & Swiss	760	296	33	6	130	1920	75	43
Arby's Turkey Club Salad (dressing not included)	350	189	21	10	90	920	9	33
Arby's Caesar Salad (dressing not included)	90	34	4	2.5	10	170	8	7
Arby's Grilled Chicken Caesar (dressing not included)	230	69	8	3.5	80	920	8	33
Arby's Chicken Finger Salad (dressing not included)	570	308	34	9	65	1300	39	30
Arby's Caesar Side Salad	45	20	2	1	5	95	4	4
Arby's Light Grilled Chicken	280	48	5	1.5	55	1170	30	29
Arby's Light Roast Chicken Deluxe	260	44	5	1	40	1010	33	23
Arby's Light Roast Turkey Deluxe	260	44	5	0.5	40	980	33	23
Arby's Roast Chicken Salad	160	21	2.5	0	40	700	15	20
Arby's Grilled Chicken Salad	210	40	4.5	1.5	65	800	14	30
Arby's Garden Salad	70	5	1	0	0	45	14	4
Arby's Side Salad	25	0	0	0	0	20	5	2
Arby's Cheddar Curly Fries	460	221	24	6	5	1290	54	6
Arby's Curly Fries (small)	310	140	15	3.5	0	770	39	4
Arby's Curly Fries (medium)	400	180	20	5	0	990	50	5
Arby's Curly Fries (large)	620	273	30	7	0	1540	78	8
Arby's Homestyle Fries (child-size)	220	86	10	2.5	0	430	32	3
Arby's Homestyle Fries (small)	300	120	13	3.5	0	570	42	3
Arby's Homestyle Fries (medium)	370	141	16	4	0	710	53	4
Arby's Homestyle Fries (large)	560	218	24	6	0	1070	79	6
Arby's Potato Cakes (2)	250	140	16	4	0	490	26	2
Arby's Jalapeno Bites	330	188	21	9	40	670	30	7
Arby's Mozzarella Sticks	470	259	29	14	60	1330	34	18
Arby's Onion Petals	410	221	24	3.5	0	300	43	4
Arby's Chicken Finger Snack	580	290	32	7	35	1450	55	19

Item								
Arby's Chicken Finger 4-Pack	640	352	38	8	70	1590	42	31
Arby's Baked Potato w/ Butter & Sour Cream	500	210	24	15	55	170	65	8
Arby's Broccoli 'N Cheddar Baked Potato	540	211	24	12	50	680	71	12
Arby's Deluxe Baked Potato	650	312	34	20	90	750	67	20
Arby's Iced Apple Turnover	420	139	16	4.5	0	230	65	4
Arby's Cherry Turnover	410	139	16	4.5	0	250	63	4
Arby's Biscuit w/ Butter	280	151	17	4	0	780	27	5
Arby's Biscuit w/ Ham	330	182	20	5	30	830	28	12
Arby's Biscuit w/ Sausage	460	299	33	9	25	300	28	12
Arby's Biscuit w/ Bacon	360	220	24	7	10	220	27	9
Arby's Croissant w/ Ham	310	171	19	11	50	1130	29	13
Arby's Croissant w/ Sausage	440	290	32	15	45	600	29	13
Arby's Croissant w/ Bacon	340	211	23	13	30	520	28	10
Arby's Sourdough w/ Ham	390	47	6	1	30	1570	67	19
Arby's Sourdough w/ Sausage	520	172	19	5	25	1040	67	19
Arby's Sourdough w/ Bacon	420	88	10	2.5	10	960	66	16
Arby's French Toastix (no syrup)	370	152	17	4	0	440	48	7
Arby's Arby's Sauce Packet	15	0	0	0	0	180	4	0
Arby's BBQ Dipping Sauce	40	0	0	0	0	350	10	0
Arby's Au Jus Sauce	5	0	.05	.02	0	386	.89	.30
Arby's BBQ Vinaigrette Dressing	140	99	11	1.5	0	660	9	0
Arby's Bleu Cheese Dressing	300	279	31	6	45	580	3	2
Arby's Bronco Berry Sauce	90	0	0	0	0	35	23	0
Arby's Buttermilk Ranch Dressing	360	349	39	6	5	490	2	1
Arby's Buttermilk Ranch Dressing Reduced Calorie	60	0	0	0	0	750	13	1
Arby's Caesar Dressing	310	310	34	5	60	470	1	1
Arby's Croutons, Cheese & Garlic	100	53	6.25	N/A	N/A	138	10	2.5
Arby's Croutons, Seasoned	30	10	1	0	0	70	5	1
Arby's German Mustard Packet	5	0	0	0	0	60	0	0

Arby's Honey French Dressing	290	209	24	4	0	410	18	0
Arby's Honey Mustard Sauce	130	111	12	1.5	10	160	5	0
Arby's Horsey Sauce Packet	60	45	5	0.5	5	150	3	0
Arby's Italian Dressing, Reduced Calorie	25	10	1	1	0	1030	3	0
Arby's Italian Parmesan Dressing	240	221	24	4	0	950	4	1
Arby's Ketchup Packet	10	0	0	0	0	100	2	0
Arby's French Toast Syrup	130	0	0	0	0	45	32	0
Arby's Mayonnaise Packet	90	90	10	1.5	10	65	0	0
Arby's Mayonnaise Packet Light, Cholesterol-Free	20	15	1.5	0	0	110	1	0
Arby's Marinara Sauce	35	12	1	0	0	260	4	1
Arby's Tangy Southwest Sauce	250	240	26	4.5	30	290	3	0
Arby's Thousand Island Dressing	290	249	28	4.5	35	480	9	1
Arby's Milk	120	43	5	3	20	120	12	8
Arby's Hot Chocolate	110	11	1	0.5	0	120	23	2
Arby's Orange Juice	140	0	0	0	0	0	34	1
Arby's Vanilla Shake	470	141	15	7	45	360	83	10
Arby's Chocolate Shake	480	149	16	8	45	370	84	10
Arby's Strawberry Shake	500	120	13	8	15	340	87	11
Arby's Jamocha Shake	470	141	15	7	45	390	82	10

Blimpie Menu	Total Calories	Fat Calories	Total Fat (g)	Sat.-rated Fat (g)	Cholest (mg)	Sodium (mg)	Carbs (g)	Protein (g)
Blimpie 6" Best Sub on White	410	120	13	5	50	1480	47	39
Blimpie 6" Best Sub on Wheat	410	120	13	5	50	1480	47	39
Blimpie 6" Cheese Trio Sub on White	490	210	23	12	55	1130	48	25
Blimpie 6" Cheese Trio Sub on Wheat	490	210	23	12	55	1110	48	26

Blimpie 6" Club Sub on White	370	90	10	4.5	30	1200	48	23
Blimpie 6" Club Sub on Wheat	370	100	11	4.5	30	1180	48	23
Blimpie 6" Ham Salami & Provolone Sub on White	480	180	20	8	55	1370	49	24
Blimpie 6" Ham Salami & Provolone Sub on Wheat	450	180	20	8	55	1350	47	24
Blimpie 6" Ham & Swiss Sub on White	410	120	14	7	50	1050	48	25
Blimpie 6" Ham & Swiss Sub on Wheat	400	130	14	7	50	1040	46	26
Blimpie 6" Tuna Sub on White	660	400	44	8	55	880	51	18
Blimpie 6" Tuna Sub on Wheat	650	400	45	6	55	860	49	18
Blimpie 6" Turkey Sub on White	330	60	6	1.5	0	1200	48	19
Blimpie 6" Turkey Sub on Wheat	330	60	7	1.5	0	1190	48	19
Blimpie 6" Roast Beef Sub on White	390	60	7	3	65	1370	47	37
Blimpie 6" Roast Beef Sub on Wheat	390	70	8	3	65	1380	45	37
Blimpie Steak & Cheese	550	230	26	3.5	70	1080	51	27
Blimpie Grilled Chicken	400	80	9	2	30	950	52	28
Blimpie Italian Meatball	500	200	22	8	25	970	52	23
Blimpie Smokey Cheddar Beef Melt	380	110	12	6	50	1200	42	23
Blimpie Roast Turkey Cordon Bleu	430	120	14	6	60	1180	43	29
Blimpie Chik Max on White	483	70	11.6	1	0	1293	69.9	33.6
Blimpie Chik Max on Wheat	495	70	12.8	1	0	1370	69.3	25.8
Blimpie Grille Max on White	413	25	6.07	1	5	823.2	71.9	18.1
Blimpie Grille Max on Wheat	425	25	7.3	1	5	900.4	71.3	18.8
Blimpie Vegi Max on White	403	30	7	0.5	0	980	61	24
Blimpie Vegi Max on Wheat	415	30	7.8	0.5	0	1050	60	24
Blimpie Mexi Max on White	393	10	4.6	1	0	1003	66	25
Blimpie Mexi Max on Wheat	405	10	5.8	1	0	1080	65	25

Item								
Blimpie Chicken Caesar Wrap	610	280	31	6	35	1770	56	26
Blimpie South Western Wrap	590	250	28	7	75	1990	56	28
Blimpie Zesty Italian Wrap	530	200	22	7	45	1850	59	24
Blimpie Antipasto Salad	200	100	11	5	50	950	9	19
Blimpie Chef Salad	150	50	6	3	40	600	8	17
Blimpie Club Salad	130	50	6	3	30	450	7	14
Blimpie Ham & Swiss Cheese Salad	170	80	8	6	40	500	7	16
Blimpie Italian Pasta Supreme Salad	180	70	7	1	0	840	20	3
Blimpie Roast Beef Salad	120	20	2.5	1.5	25	480	8	19
Blimpie Tossed Green Salad	35	5	0.5	0	0	20	7	2
Blimpie Tuna Salad	130	10	1.5	0	45	400	7	22
Blimpie Turkey Salad	90	5	0.5	0	25	580	8	15
Blimpie Cole Slaw (1/2 cup)	180	120	13	2	<5	230	13	1
Blimpie Macaroni Salad (2/3 cup)	360	220	25	4	10	660	25	4
Blimpie Mustard Potato Salad (2/3 cup)	160	45	5	1	5	660	21	2
Blimpie Potato Salad (2/3 cup)	270	170	19	3	10	560	19	2
Blimpie Classic Chili with Beans & Beef (cup)	240	70	8	3.5	40	1060	27	14
Blimpie Chicken Noodle Soup (cup)	140	30	3	1	30	1190	20	8
Blimpie Chicken Soup with White & Wild Rice (cup)	230	100	12	2	30	1210	21	10
Blimpie Cream of Potato Soup (cup)	190	80	9	2.5	<5	860	24	5
Blimpie Fat Free Italian Dressing (1 ounce)	20	0	0.0	0	0	670	5	0
Blimpie Light Italian Dressing (1.5 ounces)	20	10	1	0	0.0	810	3	0
Blimpie Light Buttermilk Ranch Dressing (1.5 ounces)	90	45	5	1	0.0	350	10	1
Blimpie Blue Cheese Dressing (1 ounce)	220	210	24	4	40	440	2	2

Blimpie Buttermilk Ranch Dressing (1 ounce)	270	260	29	4	5	360	1	0
Blimpie Honey French Dressing (1 ounce)	240	180	20	3	0.0	350	16	0
Blimpie Thousand Island Dressing (1 ounce)	210	190	21	3	25	360	7	0
Blimpie Special Sub Dressing (3/4 ounce)	70	60	7	1	0.0	0.0	0	0
Blimpie Dressing (1 ounce)	120	70	8	1	0.0	570	16	1
Blimpie Guacamole (1 ounce)	194	157.5	17.5	2.7	<1	468.1	7.4	1.8
Blimpie Mayonnaise (1 tbsp)	100	100	11.0	1.5	10.0	60	1.0	0
Blimpie Chocolate Chunk Cookie	201	90	10	6	15	201	26	2
Blimpie Macadamia White Chunk Cookie	210	90	10	5	20	140	26	2
Blimpie Oatmeal Raisin Cookie	191	70	8	2	15	201	27	3
Blimpie Peanut Butter Cookie	221	110	12	5	15	201	27	4
Blimpie Sugar Cookie	330	150	17	4.5	30	290	24.2	3
Blimpie Fudge Brownies	243.2		10.8		20	168.8	33.6	2.6
Blimpie Banana Nut Muffin	472		23		55	442	55	8
Blimpie Blueberry Muffin	412		18		55	452	55	7
Blimpie Bran & Raisin Muffin	442		18		20	502	64	7
Blimpie Cinnamon Roll	631		25		0	692	90	9
Blimpie Regular Flavored Potato Chips	210	99	11	2	0	190	25	3
Blimpie Lea & Perrins Barbecue Potato Chips	210	90	10	2	0	270	25	3
Blimpie Cheddar & Sour Cream Potato Chips	210	99	11	2	5	220	25	3
Blimpie Jalapeno Potato Chips	210	90	11	2	0	250	25	2
Blimpie Sour Cream & Onion Potato Chips	210	99	11	2	5	250	25	2
Blimpie Zesty Potato Chips	210	99	11	2	5	220	25	3

Burger King Menu	Total Calories	Fat Calories	Total Fat (g)	Sat. Fat (g)	Chol. (mg)	Sodium (mg)	Carbs (g)	Protein (g)
Burger King Biscuit	300	140	15	3.5	0	830	35	6
Burger King Cini-minis (4)	440	210	23	6	25	710	51	6
Burger King Cini-minis w/ Vanilla Icing (4)	550	235	26	6.5	25	750	71	6
Burger King French Toast Sticks (5)	390	180	20	4.5	0	440	46	6
Burger King Hash Brown Rounds (small)	240	140	15	4	0	450	23	2
Burger King Hash Brown Rounds (large)	390	230	25	7	0	760	38	3
Burger King Croissan'wich w/ Sausage, Egg & Cheese	500	320	36	13	190	1020	26	19
Burger King Croissan'wich w/ Sausage & Cheese	410	260	29	11	40	830	24	14
Burger King Biscuit w/ Egg	390	200	22	5	150	1020	37	11
Burger King Biscuit w/ Sausage	510	320	35	10	30	1190	35	13
Burger King Biscuit w/ Sausage, Egg & Cheese	650	410	46	14	190	1600	38	20
Burger King Whopper	680	350	39	12	80	940	53	29
Burger King Whopper w/ Cheese	780	420	47	17	105	1390	55	34
Burger King Double Whopper	920	510	57	20	150	1020	53	48
Burger King Double Whopper w/ Cheese	1020	590	65	25	170	1460	55	53
Burger King Whopper Jr.	410	210	23	7	50	520	32	18
Burger King Whopper Jr. w/ Cheese	460	240	27	10	60	740	33	21
Burger King Bull's-Eye BBQ Deluxe Sandwich	400	210	23	7	50	420	30	18
Burger King Hamburger	320	130	14	6	45	530	30	18
Burger King Cheeseburger	370	160	18	9	55	750	31	22
Burger King Double Hamburger	480	230	26	11	85	580	30	31
Burger King Double Cheeseburger	570	310	34	17	110	1020	32	35
Burger King Bacon Double Cheeseburger	610	330	37	18	120	1170	32	38

Item								
Burger King BK Broiler Chicken Sandwich	550	230	25	5	105	1110	52	30
Burger King Chicken Sandwich	660	350	39	8	70	1330	53	25
Burger King Chicken Tenders Sandwich	450	240	27	5	30	680	37	14
Burger King Chicken Club Sandwich	740	400	44	10	85	1530	55	30
Burger King Chicker Tenders (4)	170	80	9	3	25	420	10	11
Burger King Chicker Tenders (5)	220	110	12	3	30	530	13	14
Burger King Chicker Tenders (6)	250	130	14	4	35	630	15	16
Burger King Chicker Tenders (8)	340	170	19	5	50	840	20	22
Burger King BK Big Fish Sandwich	710	340	38	14	50	890	45	15
Burger King French Fries (small)	230	100	11	3	0	630	29	3
Burger King French Fries (medium)	360	160	18	5	0	690	46	4
Burger King French Fries (large)	500	220	25	7	0	940	63	6
Burger King French Fries (king size)	600	270	30	8	0	1140	76	7
Burger King Onion Rings (child's)	360	160	18	5	0	690	46	4
Burger King Onion Rings (medium)	320	140	16	4	0	460	40	4
Burger King Onion Rings (large)	480	210	23	6	0	690	60	7
Burger King Onion Rings (king size)	550	230	27	7	0	800	70	8
Burger King Jalapeno Poppers (4)	230	120	13	5	20	790	22	7
Burger King Mozarella Sticks (4)	290	140	16	6	20	670	25	12
Burger King Dutch Apple Pie	340	130	14	3	3	470	52	2
Burger King Hershey's Sundae Pie	310	160	18	13	10	130	35	3
Burger King Vanilla Shake (small)	330	50	6	4	20	260	61	9

Item								
Burger King Vanilla Shake (medium)	430	70	8	5	25	340	79	12
Burger King Chocolate Shake w/ Syrup (small)	400	50	6	4	20	360	77	10
Burger King Chocolate Shake w/ Syrup (medium)	500	70	8	5	25	440	95	13
Burger King Strawberry Shake w/ Syrup (small)	390	50	6	4	20	270	76	9
Burger King Strawberry Shake w/ Syrup (medium)	500	70	8	5	25	350	95	12
Burger King Coca Cola Classic (small)	160	0	0	0	0		41	0
Burger King Coca Cola Classic (medium)	230	0	0	0	0		56	0
Burger King Coca Cola Classic (large)	330	0	0	0	0		82	0
Burger King Coca Cola Classic (king)	430	0	0	0	0		108	0
Burger King Diet Coke (small)	0	0	0	0	0		0	0
Burger King Diet Coke (medium)	0	0	0	0	0		0	0
Burger King Diet Coke (large)	0	0	0	0	0		0	0
Burger King Diet Coke (king)	0	0	0	0	0		0	0
Burger King Sprite (small)	160	0	0	0	0		40	0
Burger King Sprite (medium)	220	0	0	0	0		55	0
Burger King Sprite (large)	320	0	0	0	0		80	0
Burger King Sprite (king)	420	0	0	0	0		105	0
Burger King Dr. Pepper (small)	160	0	0	0	0		39	0
Burger King Dr. Pepper (medium)	220	0	0	0	0		54	0
Burger King Dr. Pepper (large)	320	0	0	0	0		79	0
Burger King Dr. Pepper (king)	410	0	0	0	0		104	0
Burger King Frozen Coca Cola Classic (medium)	370	0	0	0	0		92	0
Burger King Frozen Coca Cola Classic (large)	460	0	0	0	0		116	0
Burger King Frozen Minute Maid Cherry (medium)	370	0	0	0	0		92	0
Burger King Frozen Minute Maid Cherry (large)	460	0	0	0	0		116	0

	Total Calories	Fat Calories	Total Fat (g)	Sat. Fat (g)	Chol. (mg)	Sodium (mg)	Carbs (g)	Protein (g)
Burger King Coffee (small)	0	0	0	0	0	0	0	0
Burger King Coffee (medium)	5	0	0	0	0	5	0	0
Burger King Coffee (large)	10	0	0	0	0	10	0	0
Burger King Tropicana Pure Orange Juice	140	0	0	0	0	0	33	2
Burger King Milk (2% fat)	130	45	5	3	20	120	12	8

* a suggested serving size of 1 slice

Carl's Jr. Menu	Total Calories	Fat Calories	Total Fat (g)	Sat. Fat (g)	Chol. (mg)	Sodium (mg)	Carbs (g)	Protein (g)
Carl's Jr. Carl's Famous Star	590	290	32	9	70	910	50	24
Carl's Jr. Super Star	790	420	47	15	130	980	51	41
Carl's Jr. Sourdough Bacon Cheeseburger	640	370	41	15	95	690	37	30
Carl's Jr. Sourdough Ranch Bacon Cheeseburger	720	410	46	16	95	800	43	33
Carl's Jr. Double Sourdough Bacon Cheeseburger	880	530	59	24	165	1010	37	50
Carl's Jr. Western Bacon Cheeseburger	660	270	30	12	85	1410	64	31
Carl's Jr. Double Western Bacon Cheeseburger	920	450	50	21	155	1770	65	51
Carl's Jr. Famous Bacon Cheeseburger	700	370	41	13	95	1310	51	31
Carl's Jr. Hamburger	280	80	9	3.5	35	480	36	14
Carl's Jr. Charbroiled BBQ Chicken Sandwich	290	30	3.5	1	60	840	41	25
Carl's Jr. Charbroiled BBQ Club Sandwich	470	200	23	7	95	1110	37	31
Carl's Jr. Charbroiled Santa Fe Chicken Sandwich	540	280	31	8	95	1210	37	28
Carl's Jr. Ranch Crispy Chicken Sandwich	660	280	31	7	70	1180	71	24
Carl's Jr. Bacon Swiss Crispy Chicken Sandwich	760	350	38	11	90	1550	72	31
Carl's Jr. Western Bacon Crispy Chicken Sandwich	750	250	28	11	80	1900	91	31
Carl's Jr. Spicy Chicken Sandwich	480	230	26	5	40	1220	47	14

Carl's Jr.	Total Calories	Fat Calories	Total Fat (g)	Sat. Fat (g)	Chol. (mg)	Sodium (mg)	Carbs (g)	Protein (g)
Carl's Jr. Southwest Spicy Chicken Sandwich	620	370	41	10	65	1640	48	16
Carl's Jr. Charbroiled Sirloin Steak Sandwich	550	220	24	4.5	80	1080	52	30
Carl's Jr. Carl's Catch Fish Sandwich	530	250	28	7	80	1030	55	18
Carl's Jr. American Cheese (large)	60	45	5	3.5	15	260	1	3
Carl's Jr. American Cheese (small)	50	35	4	2.5	10	200	1	3
Carl's Jr. Swiss-Style Cheese	50	35	4	2.5	15	230	0	4
Carl's Jr. French Fries (kids)	250	110	12	2.5	0	150	32	4
Carl's Jr. French Fries (small)	290	120	14	3	0	180	37	5
Carl's Jr. French Fries (medium)	460	200	22	5	0	280	59	7
Carl's Jr. French Fries (large)	620	260	29	6	0	380	80	10
Carl's Jr. Onion Rings	430	190	22	5	0	700	53	7
Carl's Jr. Zucchini	320	170	19	5	0	860	31	6
Carl's Jr. Hash Brown Nuggets	330	190	21	4.5	0	470	32	3
Carl's Jr. Crisscut Fries	410	220	24	5	0	950	43	5
Carl's Jr. Chicken Stars (6 pieces)	260	150	16	4.5	40	480	14	13

Church's Chicken Menu	Total Calories	Fat Calories	Total Fat (g)	Sat. Fat (g)	Chol. (mg)	Sodium (mg)	Carbs (g)	Protein (g)
Church's Chicken Wing	250	145	16		60	540	7.7	18.5
Church's Chicken Leg	250	82	9.1		45	160	2.4	12.7
Church's Chicken Thigh	230	146	16.2		80	520	16.2	16.2
Church's Chicken Breast	200	111	12.4		65	510	19	19
Church's Chicken Tender Strip	80	36	4		15	140	6	6
Church's Cajun Rice (3.1 ounces)	130	63	7		5	260	15.6	1.3
Church's Mashed Potatoes & Gravy (3.7 ounces)	90	29.7	3.3		0	520	14	1.2
Church's Okra (2.8 ounces)	210	145	16.1		0	520	19.1	2.7
Church's Corn On The Cob (5.7 ounces)	139	29	3.2		0	15	23.5	4.4

	Total Calories	Fat Calories	Total Fat (g)	Sat. Fat (g)	Chol. (mg)	Sodium (mg)	Carbs (g)	Protein (g)
Church's Cole Slaw (3 ounces)	92	49.5	5.5	0	230	8.4	4.2	
Church's French Fries (2.7 ounces)	210	94.5	10.5	0	60	28.5	3.3	
Church's Macaroni & Cheese (3.6 ounces)	140	60	7	10	460	15	5	
Church's Jalapeño Bombers (5 ounces)	300	108	12	35	1210	36	10	
Church's Honey Butter Biscuits (2.1 ounces)	250	147.5	16.4	5	640	25.6	2.2	
Church's Apple Pie (3.1 ounces)	280	110.7	12.3	5	340	40.5	2.3	

Dairy Queen Menu	Total Calories	Fat Calories	Total Fat (g)	Sat. Fat (g)	Chol. (mg)	Sodium (mg)	Carbs (g)	Protein (g)
Dairy Queen DQ Homestyle Hamburger	290	110	12	5	45	630	29	17
Dairy Queen DQ Homestyle Cheeseburger	340	150	17	8	55	850	29	20
Dairy Queen DQ Homestyle Double Cheeseburger	540	280	31	16	115	1130	30	35
Dairy Queen DQ Homestyle Bacon Double Cheeseburger	610	320	36	18	130	1380	31	41
Dairy Queen DQ Ultimate Burger	670	390	43	19	135	1210	29	40
Dairy Queen Hot Dog	240	120	14	5	25	730	19	9
Dairy Queen Chili 'n' Cheese Dog	330	190	21	9	45	1090	22	14
Dairy Queen Chicken Breast Fillet Sandwich	430	180	20	4	55	760	37	24
Dairy Queen Grilled Chicken Sandwich	310	90	10	2.5	50	1040	30	24
Dairy Queen Chicken Strip Basket	1000	450	50	13	55	2510	102	35
Dairy Queen The Great Steakmelt Basket	770	340	38	13	75	2290	72	32
Dairy Queen French Fries (small)	350	160	18	3.5	0	880	42	4
Dairy Queen French Fries (medium)	440	200	23	4.5	0	1110	53	5
Dairy Queen Onion Rings	320	140	16	4	0	180	39	5

Domino's Pizza Menu	Total Calories	Fat Calories	Total Fat (g)	Sat. Fat (g)	Chol. (mg)	Sodium (mg)	Carbs (g)	Protein (g)
Domino's Pizza Classic Hand Tossed 12" Cheese*	375		11	5	23	776	55	21
Domino's Pizza Classic Hand Tossed 14" Cheese*	516		15	7	32	1080	75	21
Domino's Pizza Crunchy Thin Crust 12" Cheese*	273		12	5	23	835	31	12
Domino's Pizza Crunchy Thin Crust 14" Cheese*	382		17	7	32	1172	43	17
Domino's Pizza Ultimate Deep Dish 6" Cheese	598		28	10	36	1341	68	23
Domino's Pizza Ultimate Deep Dish 12" Cheese*	482		22	8	30	1123	56	19
Domino's Pizza Ultimate Deep Dish 14" Cheese*	677		30	11	41	1575	80	26

* a suggested serving size of 2 slices

Dunkin' Donuts Menu	Total Calories	Fat Calories	Total Fat (g)	Sat. Fat (g)	Chol. (mg)	Sodium (mg)	Carbs (g)	Protein (g)
Dunkin' Donuts Apple Crumb Donut	230	90	10	3	0	270	34	3
Dunkin' Donuts Apple Fritter	300	130	14	3	0	360	41	4
Dunkin' Donuts Apple N' Spice Donut	200	70	8	1.5	0	270	29	3
Dunkin' Donuts Bavarian Kreme Donut	210	80	9	2	0	270	30	3
Dunkin' Donuts Chocolate Iced Donut	340	130	15	3.5	0	290	50	3
Dunkin' Donuts Black Raspberry Donut	210	70	8	1.5	0	280	32	3
Dunkin' Donuts Blueberry Cake Donut	290	150	16	3.5	10	400	35	3
Dunkin' Donuts Blueberry Crumb Donut	240	90	10	3	0	260	36	3
Dunkin' Donuts Boston Kreme Donut	240	80	9	2	0	280	36	3
Dunkin' Donuts Bow Tie Donut	300	150	17	3.5	0	340	34	4

Dunkin' Donuts Butternut Cake Donut Ring	300	150	16	4.5	0	360	36	3
Dunkin' Donuts Caramel Apple Krunch Donut	300	130	14	3	0	310	41	4
Dunkin' Donuts Chocolate Coconut Cake Donut	300	170	19	6	0	370	31	4
Dunkin' Donuts Chocolate Frosted Cake Donut	300	140	16	3	0	370	38	3
Dunkin' Donuts Chocolate Frosted Coffee Roll	290	130	15	3	0	340	36	4
Dunkin' Donuts Chocolate Frosted Donut	200	80	9	2	0	260	29	3
Dunkin' Donuts Chocolate Glazed Cake Donut	290	150	16	3.5	0	370	33	3
Dunkin' Donuts Chocolate Kreme Filled Donut	270	110	13	3	0	260	35	3
Dunkin' Donuts Cinnamon Bun	510	140	15	4	10	420	85	8
Dunkin' Donuts Cinnamon Cake Donut	270	130	15	3	0	360	31	3
Dunkin' Donuts Coconut Cake Donut	290	150	17	5	0	360	33	3
Dunkin' Donuts Coffee Roll	270	130	14	3	0	340	33	4
Dunkin' Donuts Double Chocolate Cake Donut	310	160	17	3.5	0	370	37	3
Dunkin' Donuts Dunkin' Donut	240	130	15	3	0	340	25	3
Dunkin' Donuts Eclair Donut	270	100	11	2.5	0	290	39	3
Dunkin' Donuts Glazed Cake Donut	270	130	15	3	0	360	33	3
Dunkin' Donuts Glazed Chocolate Cruller	280	130	15	3	0	360	35	3
Dunkin' Donuts Glazed Cruller	290	130	15	3	0	350	37	3
Dunkin' Donuts Glazed Donut	180	70	8	1.5	0	250	25	3
Dunkin' Donuts Glazed Fritter	260	130	14	3	0	330	31	4
Dunkin' Donuts Jelly Filled Donut	210	70	8	1.5	0	280	32	3
Dunkin' Donuts Jelly Stick	290	110	12	2.5	0	390	44	3
Dunkin' Donuts Lemon Donut	200	80	9	2	0	270	28	3
Dunkin' Donuts Maple Frosted Coffee Roll	290	130	14	3	0	340	36	4

Dunkin' Donuts Maple Frosted Donut	210	80	9	2	0	260	30	3
Dunkin' Donuts Marble Frosted Donut	200	80	9	2	0	260	29	3
Dunkin' Donuts Old Fashioned Cake Donut	250	140	15	3	0	360	26	3
Dunkin' Donuts Plain Cruller	240	130	15	3	0	340	25	3
Dunkin' Donuts Powdered Cake Donut	270	140	15	3	0	350	32	3
Dunkin' Donuts Powdered Cruller	270	130	15	3	0	340	30	3
Dunkin' Donuts Strawberry Donut	210	70	8	1.5	0	260	32	3
Dunkin' Donuts Strawberry Frosted Donut	210	80	9	2	0	260	30	3
Dunkin' Donuts Sugar Cruller	250	130	15	3	0	340	27	3
Dunkin' Donuts Sugar Raised Donut	170	70	8	1.5	0	250	22	3
Dunkin' Donuts Sugared Cake Donut	250	130	15	3	0	350	27	3
Dunkin' Donuts Toasted Coconut Cake Donut	300	150	17	5	0	370	35	3
Dunkin' Donuts Vanilla Frosted Coffee Roll	290	130	14	3	0	340	36	4
Dunkin' Donuts Vanilla Frosted Donut	210	80	9	2	0	260	30	3
Dunkin' Donuts Vanilla Kreme Filled Donut	270	110	13	3	0	250	36	3
Dunkin' Donuts Whole Wheat Glazed Cake Donut	310	170	19	4	0	380	32	4
Dunkin' Donuts Butternut Cake Munchkins (3)	200	100	11	3	0	240	25	2
Dunkin' Donuts Cinnamon Cake Munchkins (3)	250	130	14	3	0	330	30	3
Dunkin' Donuts Coconut Cake Munchkins (3)	200	100	12	3.5	0	240	23	2
Dunkin' Donuts Glazed Cake Munchkins (3)	200	90	10	2	0	250	27	2
Dunkin' Donuts Plain Cake Munchkins (3)	220	120	14	3	0	310	22	2
Dunkin' Donuts Powdered Cake Munchkins (3)	250	130	14	3	0	310	29	2

Dunkin' Donuts Sugared Cake Munchkins (3)	240	120	14	3	0	310	28	2
Dunkin' Donuts Toasted Coconut Cake Munchkins (3)	200	100	11	3	0	250	24	2
Dunkin' Donuts Glazed Chocolate Cake Munchkins (3)	200	90	10	2	0	250	26	2
Dunkin' Donuts Glazed Yeast Munchkins (3)	200	80	9	2	0	220	27	3
Dunkin' Donuts Jelly Filled Yeast Munchkins (3)	210	80	9	2	0	240	30	3
Dunkin' Donuts Lemon Filled Yeast Munchkins (3)	170	70	8	1.5	0	190	23	2
Dunkin' Donuts Sugar Raised Yeast Munchkins (3)	220	110	12	2.5	0	290	26	4
Dunkin' Donuts Berry Berry Bagel	340	25	3	0.5	0	540	69	11
Dunkin' Donuts Blueberry Bagel	340	25	3	0.5	0	630	69	11
Dunkin' Donuts Cinnamon Raisin Bagel	340	30	3.5	0.5	0	600	69	11
Dunkin' Donuts Everything Bagel	360	25	2.5	0.5	0	710	67	12
Dunkin' Donuts Garlic Bagel	360	25	2.5	0.5	0	720	68	12
Dunkin' Donuts Onion Bagel	350	35	4	1	0	660	66	12
Dunkin' Donuts Plain Bagel	340	25	2.5	0.5	0	680	67	12
Dunkin' Donuts Poppyseed Bagel	360	35	4	0.5	0	710	68	12
Dunkin' Donuts Salt Bagel	340	25	2.5	0.5	0	3030	67	12
Dunkin' Donuts Sesame Bagel	380	40	4.5	0.5	0	720	74	12
Dunkin' Donuts Sundried Tomato Bagel	330	25	2.5	0.5	0	700	66	13
Dunkin' Donuts Wheat Bagel	350	40	4.5	1	0	640	67	13
Dunkin' Donuts Chive Cream Cheese*	190	170	19	13	55	220	3	3
Dunkin' Donuts Garden Vegetable Cream Cheese*	180	160	17	11	45	310	3	3
Dunkin' Donuts Lite Cream Cheese*	130	100	11	7	30	250	3	5
Dunkin' Donuts Plain Cream Cheese*	200	170	19	13	60	230	3	4

Item								
Dunkin' Donuts Salmon Cream Cheese*	180	150	17	11	50	150	2	5
Dunkin' Donuts Strawberry Cream Cheese*	180	145	16	9	0	170	9	2
Dunkin' Donuts Apple Cinnamon Pecan Muffin	510	190	21	6	70	590	74	8
Dunkin' Donuts Banana Nut Muffin	530	200	23	6	75	540	72	10
Dunkin' Donuts Blueberry Muffin	490	160	17	6	75	610	76	8
Dunkin' Donuts Chocolate Chip Muffin	590	210	24	10	75	560	88	9
Dunkin' Donuts Corn Muffin	500	150	16	4.5	80	920	78	10
Dunkin' Donuts Cranberry Orange Muffin	470	140	15	5	75	600	76	8
Dunkin' Donuts Honey Bran Raisin Muffin	490	140	16	3.5	30	880	84	7
Dunkin' Donuts Lemon Poppyseed Muffin	580	170	19	6	85	620	94	10
Dunkin' Donuts Reduced Fat Blueberry Muffin	450	110	12	9	65	590	77	8
Dunkin' Donuts Biscuit	280	130	14	4	0	850	32	6
Dunkin' Donuts Plain Croissant	290	160	18	6	5	270	26	5
Dunkin' Donuts Bagel Bacon Cheddar Omwich	600	190	21	8	295	1630	79	26
Dunkin' Donuts Bagel Pizza Omwich	560	165	19	6	255	1305	74	25
Dunkin' Donuts Bagel Spanish Omwich	570	160	18	6	280	1370	79	24
Dunkin' Donuts Biscuit Bacon Cheddar Omwich	500	290	32	11	300	1660	33	21
Dunkin' Donuts Biscuit Egg & Cheese Sandwich	380	200	22	8	180	1250	30	17
Dunkin' Donuts Biscuit Pizza Omwich	500	270	30	9	255	1475	39	19
Dunkin' Donuts Biscuit Sausage, Egg & Cheese Sandwich	590	370	42	15	220	1620	31	25
Dunkin' Donuts Biscuit Spanish Omwich	470	260	29	9	285	1400	34	19
Dunkin' Donuts Croissant Bacon Cheddar Omwich	560	350	38	13	295	1190	33	21

114

Dunkin' Donuts Croissant Pizza Omwich	510	300	34	11	260	895	33	18
Dunkin' Donuts Croissant Spanish Cheese Omwich	530	320	36	11	285	930	33	19
Dunkin' Donuts English Muffin Bacon Cheddar Omwich	400	190	21	8	295	1440	33	21
Dunkin' Donuts English Muffin Ham, Egg & Cheese	320	110	12	6	195	1340	31	22
Dunkin' Donuts English Muffin Pizza Omwich	350	150	17	6	255	1145	33	17
Dunkin' Donuts English Muffin Spanish Omwich	370	160	18	6	280	1180	34	18
Dunkin' Donuts Chocolate Chocolate Chunk Cookie	210	100	11	7	35	110	26	3
Dunkin' Donuts Chocolate Chunk Cookie	220	100	11	7	35	105	28	3
Dunkin' Donuts Chocolate Chunk Cookie w/ Nuts	230	110	12	6	35	110	27	3
Dunkin' Donuts Chocolate-White Chocolate Chunk Cookie	230	110	12	7	35	120	28	3
Dunkin' Donuts Oatmeal Raisin Pecan Cookie	220	90	10	5	30	110	29	3
Dunkin' Donuts Peanut Butter Chocolate Chunk Cookie w/ Nuts	240	130	14	6	25	125	24	4
Dunkin' Donuts Peanut Butter Cookie w/ Nuts	240	130	14	6	30	150	24	5
Dunkin' Donuts Coffee Coolatta w/ Cream	410	200	22	14	75	65	51	3
Dunkin' Donuts Coffee Coolatta w/ 2% Milk	240	20	2	1.5	10	80	52	4
Dunkin' Donuts Coffee Coolatta w/ Cream & Chocolate Mint Cookie Coolatta Whirl-Ins	460	220	24	14	75	120	58	4
Dunkin' Donuts Coffee Coolatta w/ Cream & Coolatta Whirl-Ins made with Oreo Cookie	460	210	24	14	75	150	58	4
Dunkin' Donuts Coffee Coolatta w/ Milk	260	35	4	2.5	15	75	52	4
Dunkin' Donuts Coffee Coolatta w/ Milk & Chocolate Mint Cookie Coolatta Whirl-Ins	310	50	6	3	15	130	59	4

	Total Calories	Fat Calories	Total Fat (g)	Sat. Fat (g)	Chol. (mg)	Sodium (mg)	Carbs (g)	Protein (g)
Dunkin' Donuts Coffee Coolatta w/ Milk & Coolatta Whirl-Ins made with Oreo Cookie	300	50	5	3	15	160	60	4
Dunkin' Donuts Coffee Coolatta w/ Skim Milk	230	0	0	0	5	80	52	4
Dunkin' Donuts Coffee Coolatta w/ Skim Milk & Chocolate Mint Cookie Coolatta Whirl-Ins	280	20	2.5	0	5	135	59	4
Dunkin' Donuts Coffee Coolatta w/ Skim Milk & Coolatta Whirl-Ins made with Oreo Cookie	270	15	2	0	5	160	60	5
Dunkin' Donuts Dunkaccino	250	100	11	3.5	10	240	34	2
Dunkin' Donuts Hot Chocolate	230	70	8	2	0	310	38	2
Dunkin' Donuts Orange Mango Fruit Coolatta	290	0	0	0	0	30	71	1
Dunkin' Donuts Pina Coolatta	270	30	3.5	3	0	65	57	1
Dunkin' Donuts Strawberry Fruit Coolatta	280	0	0	0	0	30	70	0
Dunkin' Donuts Vanilla Bean Coolatta	450	70	7	4	0	170	94	1
Dunkin' Donuts Vanilla Bean Coolatta & Coolatta Whirl-Ins made with Oreo Cookie	500	160	18	15	0	170	83	2
Dunkin' Donuts Vanilla Bean Coolatta w/ Chocolate Mint Cookie Coolatta Whirl-Ins	500	170	19	15	0	150	82	2

* a suggested serving size of 1 packet

In-N-Out Burger Menu	Total Calories	Fat Calories	Total Fat (g)	Sat. Fat (g)	Chol. (mg)	Sodium (mg)	Carbs (g)	Protein (g)
In-N-Out Burger Hamburger	390	170	19	5	40	640	39	16
In-N-Out Burger Cheeseburger	480	240	27	10	60	1000	39	22
In-N-Out Burger Double-Double	670	370	41	18	120	1430	40	37
In-N-Out Burger French Fries	400	160	18	5	0	245	54	7
In-N-Out Burger Chocolate Shake	690	320	36	24	95	350	83	9
In-N-Out Burger Vanilla Shake	680	330	37	25	90	390	78	9
In-N-Out Burger Strawberry Shake	690	300	33	22	85	280	91	8

	Total Calories	Fat Calories	Total Fat (g)	Sa. Fat (g)	Chol. (mg)	Sodium (mg)	Carbs (g)	Protein (g)
In-N-Out Burger Coca-Cola Classic	198	0	0	0	0	12	54	0
In-N-Out Burger Diet Coca-Cola	0	0	0	0	0	20	0	0
In-N-Out Burger Seven-Up	220	0	0	0	0	40	52	0
In-N-Out Burger Dr. Pepper	200	0	0	0	0	0	52	0
In-N-Out Burger Root Beer	222	0	0	0	0	48	60	0
In-N-Out Burger Lemonade	180	0	0	0	0	20	40	0
In-N-Out Burger Iced Tea	0	0	0	0	0	0	0	0
In-N-Out Burger Coffee	5	0	0	0	0	3	1	0
In-N-Out Burger Milk	180	50	6	4	30	190	18	12

Jack In The Box Menu	Total Calories	Fat Calories	Total Fat (g)	Sa. Fat (g)	Chol. (mg)	Sodium (mg)	Carbs (g)	Protein (g)
Jack In The Box Bacon	20	10	1.5	0.5	5	95	0	2
Jack In The Box Biscuit	190	80	9	2.5	0	500	24	3
Jack In The Box French Toast Sticks	420	180	20	4	5	420	53	7
Jack In The Box Hash Browns	170	110	12	2	0	250	14	1
Jack In The Box Ultimate Cheeseburger	950	590	66	26	195	1370	37	52
Jack In The Box Bacon Ultimate Cheeseburger	1020	640	71	26	210	1740	37	58
Jack In The Box Sourdough Jack	690	410	45	15	105	1180	37	34
Jack In The Box Bacon Bacon Cheeseburger	760	450	50	17	135	1570	39	39
Jack In The Box Jumbo Jack	550	270	30	10	75	880	43	27
Jack In The Box Jumbo Jack w/ Cheese	640	340	38	15	105	1340	44	31
Jack In The Box Double Cheeseburger	440	220	24	11	80	1100	31	24
Jack In The Box Hamburger	250	80	9	3.5	30	610	30	12
Jack In The Box Hamburger w/ Cheese	300	120	13	6	40	840	31	14
Jack In The Box Jack's Spicy Chicken	570	260	29	2.5	50	1020	52	24
Jack In The Box Chicken Fajita Pita	320	90	10	4.5	55	850	34	24

Jack In The Box Grilled Chicken Fillet	480	220	24	6	65	1110	39	27
Jack In The Box Chicken Supreme	830	440	49	7	65	2140	66	33
Jack In The Box Chicken Sandwich	400	180	21	3	40	770	38	15
Jack In The Box Chicken Breast Pieces (5)	360	150	17	3	80	970	24	27
Jack In The Box Sourdough Grilled Chicken Club	520	240	27	6	80	1320	39	31
Jack In The Box Fish & Chips	780	350	39	9	45	1740	86	19
Jack In The Box Chicken Teriyaki Bowl	670	40	4	1	15	1730	128	26
Jack In The Box Taco	170	90	10	3.5	15	390	12	7
Jack In The Box Monster Taco	270	150	17	6	30	630	19	12
Jack In The Box Garden Chicken Salad	200	80	9	4	65	420	8	23
Jack In The Box Side Salad	50	30	3	1.5	10	75	3	2
Jack In The Box French Fries (regular)	350	150	16	4	0	710	46	4
Jack In The Box French Fries (jumbo)	430	180	20	5	0	890	58	4
Jack In The Box French Fries (super scoop)	610	260	28	6	0	1250	82	6
Jack In The Box Seasoned Curly Fries	410	210	23	5	0	1010	45	6
Jack In The Box Onion Rings	450	230	25	5	0	780	50	7
Jack In The Box Chili Cheese Curly Fries	650	370	41	12	25	1760	60	14
Jack In The Box Bacon Cheddar Potato Wedges	750	450	50	16	45	1510	55	20
Jack In The Box Stuffed Jalapeños (3)	230	120	13	5	25	740	20	7
Jack In The Box Stuffed Jalapeños (7)	530	280	31	12	60	1730	46	16
Jack In The Box Egg Roll	150	70	8	2	10	340	13	5
Jack In The Box Egg Rolls (3)	440	220	24	6	30	1020	40	15
Jack In The Box Cheesecake	320	160	18	10	65	220	32	7
Jack In The Box Double Fudge Cake	300	90	10	2	50	320	50	3

	Total Calories	Fat Calories	Total Fat (g)	Sat. Fat (g)	Chol. (mg)	Sodium (mg)	Carbs (g)	Protein (g)
Jack In The Box Hot Apple Turnover	340	160	18	4	0	510	85	4
Jack In The Box Oreo Cookie Shake (regular)	740	320	36	19	95	490	91	13
Jack In The Box Cappuccino Shake (regular)	630	260	29	17	90	320	80	11
Jack In The Box Chocolate Shake (regular)	630	240	27	16	85	330	85	11
Jack In The Box Strawberry Shake (regular)	640	250	28	15	85	300	85	10
Jack In The Box Vanilla Shake (regular)	610	280	31	18	95	320	73	12
Jack In The Box Coca Cola Classic (regular)	170	0	0	0	0		46	0
Jack In The Box Diet Coke (regular)	0	0	0	0	0	15	0	0
Jack In The Box Sprite (regular)	160	0	0	0	0	40	41	0
Jack In The Box Dr. Pepper (regular)	190	0	0	0	0	25	49	0
Jack In The Box Barq's Root Beer (regular)	180	0	0	0	0	40	50	0
Jack In The Box Minute Maid Lemonade (regular)	190	0	0	0	0	100	65	0
Jack In The Box Coffee (regular)	5	0	0	0	0	5	1	0
Jack In The Box Orange Juice	150	0	0	0	0	20	34	2
Jack In The Box Milk (2% fat)	130	45	5	3	25	85	14	9

Kentucky Fried Chicken Menu	Total Calories	Fat Calories	Total Fat (g)	Sat. Fat (g)	Chol. (mg)	Sodium (mg)	Carbs (g)	Protein (g)
KFC Original Recipe Chicken Wing	140	90	10	2.5	55	414	5	9
KFC Original Recipe Chicken Breast	400	220	24	6	135	1116	16	29
KFC Original Recipe Chicken Drumstick	140	80	9	2	75	422	4	13
KFC Original Recipe Chicken Thigh	250	160	18	4.5	95	747	6	16
KFC Extra Crispy Chicken Wing	220	140	15	4	55	415	10	10
KFC Extra Crispy Chicken Breast	470	240	28	8	160	874	17	39

KFC Extra Crispy Chicken Drumstick	195	110	12	3	77	375	7	15
KFC Extra Crispy Chicken Thigh	380	250	27	7	118	625	14	21
KFC Hot & Spicy Chicken Wing	210	130	25	4	55	350	9	10
KFC Hot & Spicy Chicken Breast	505	270	29	8	162	1170	23	38
KFC Hot & Spicy Chicken Drumstick	175	90	10	3	77	360	9	13
KFC Hot & Spicy Chicken Thigh	355	225	26	7	126	630	13	19
KFC Original Recipe Sandwich w/ Sauce	450	200	22	5	70	940	33	29
KFC Original Recipe Sandwich (no sauce)	360	120	13	3.5	60	890	21	29
KFC Triple Crunch Sandwich w/ Sauce	490	260	29	6	70	710	39	28
KFC Triple Crunch Sandwich (no sauce)	390	140	15	4.5	50	650	29	25
KFC Triple Crunch Zinger Sandwich w/ Sauce	550	290	32	7	85	830	39	28
KFC Triple Crunch Zinger Sandwich (no sauce)	390	140	15	4.5	50	650	36	25
KFC Tender Roast Sandwich w/ Sauce	350	130	15	3	75	880	26	32
KFC Tender Roast Sandwich (no sauce)	270	45	5	1.5	65	690	23	31
KFC Honey BBQ Flavored Sandwich w/ Sauce	310	50	6	2	125	560	37	28
KFC Colonel's Crispy Strips (3)	300	125	16	4	56	1165	18	26
KFC Spicy Crispy Strips (3)	335	140	15	4	70	1140	23	25
KFC Popcorn Chicken (small)	362	207	23	6	43	610	21	17
KFC Popcorn Chicken (large)	620	356	40	10	73	1046	36	30
KFC Chunky Chicken Pot Pie	770	378	42	13	70	2160	69	29
KFC Hot Wings Pieces (6)	471	297	33	8	150	1230	18	27
KFC Honey BBQ Pieces (6)	607	343	38	10	193	1145	33	33
KFC Mashed Potatoes w/ Gravy (4.8 ounces)	120	50	6	1	1	440	17	1
KFC Potato Wedges	280	120	13	4	5	750	28	5
KFC Macaroni & Cheese (5.4 ounces)	180	70	8	3	10	860	21	7

	Total Calories	Fat Calories	Total Fat (g)	Sat. Fat (g)	Chol. (mg)	Sodium (mg)	Carbs (g)	Protein (g)
KFC Corn On The Cob	150	15	1.5	0	0	20	35	5
KFC BBQ Baked Beans (5.5 ounces)	190	25	3	1	5	760	33	6
KFC Cole Slaw (5 ounces)	232	121	13.5	2	8	284	26	2
KFC Cole Slaw (5.6 ounces)	230	130	14	2	15	540	23	4
KFC Biscuit	180	80	10	2.5	0	560	20	4
KFC Double Chocolate Chip Cake	320	140	16	4	55	230	41	4
KFC Fudge Brownie Parfait	280	90	10	3.5	145	190	44	3
KFC Lemon Creme Parfait	410	130	14	8	20	290	62	7
KFC Chocolate Creme Parfait	290	130	15	11	15	330	37	3
KFC Strawberry Shortcake Parfait	200	60	7	6	10	220	33	1
KFC Twister	600	300	34	7	50	1430	52	22
KFC Honey BBQ Crunch Melt	556	235	26	5	60	1010	48	33
KFC Pecan Pie*	490	200	23	5	65	510	66	5
KFC Apple Pie*	310	130	14	3	0	280	44	2
KFC Strawberry Creme Pie*	280	130	15	8	15	130	32	4

* a suggested serving size of 1 slice

Krispy Kreme Doughnuts Menu	Total Calories	Fat Calories	Total Fat (g)	Sat. Fat (g)	Chol. (mg)	Sodium (mg)	Carbs (g)	Protein (g)
Krispy Kreme Original Glazed	210	110	12	4	4.5	65	22	2
Krispy Kreme Fudge Iced Glazed	280	130	14	4	4.5	75	36	3
Krispy Kreme Fudge Iced Sprinkles	220	90	10	2.5	4.5	95	31	2
Krispy Kreme Maple Iced Glazed	200	80	9	2.5	0	100	28	3
Krispy Kreme Cinnamon Apple Filled	280	120	13	3	4.5	180	35	5
Krispy Kreme Powdered Blueberry Filled	270	110	13	4	4.5	170	33	5
Krispy Kreme Fudge Iced Creme Filled	340	160	18	5	4.5	160	39	5

	Calories	Fat Calories	Total Fat (g)	Sat. Fat (g)	Chol. (mg)	Sodium (mg)	Carbs (g)	Protein (g)
Krispy Kreme Fudge Iced Custard Filled	310	140	16	4	4.5	170	39	4
Krispy Kreme Glazed Raspberry Filled	270	110	12	3	4.5	170	37	4
Krispy Kreme Glazed Lemon Filled	280	130	14	4	4.5	160	33	5
Krispy Kreme Glazed Creme Filled	350	120	20	5	4.5	135	39	4
Krispy Kreme Traditional Cake	200	100	11	3	15	280	22	3
Krispy Kreme Cinnamon Twist	220	100	11	3	5	150	27	4
Krispy Kreme Fudge Iced Cake	230	110	12	3	15	280	28	3
Krispy Kreme Glazed Cruller	250	140	16	4	5	190	24	2
Krispy Kreme Fudge Iced Glazed Cruller	240	110	12	3	10	160	31	2
Krispy Kreme Glazed Devil's Food	390	220	24	5	4.5	250	41	2
Krispy Kreme Cinnamon Bun	220	100	11	3	0	160	26	5
Krispy Kreme Glazed Blueberry	300	140	15	3	5	200	37	2

Little Caesar's Menu	Total Calories	Fat Calories	Total Fat (g)	Sat. Fat (g)	Chol. (mg)	Sodium (mg)	Carbs (g)	Protein (g)
Little Caesar's 12" Round Cheese Pizza*	160		6	2.5	15	320	22	8
Little Caesar's 12" Round Pepperoni Pizza*	180		8	3	20	420	21	9
Little Caesar's 14" Round Cheese Pizza*	170		6	2.5	15	360	23	8
Little Caesar's 14" Round Pepperoni Pizza*	200		8	3.5	20	460	23	9
Little Caesar's 14" Round Supreme Pizza*	230		10	4	25	550	25	11
Little Caesar's 14" Round Meatsa Pizza*	220		10	4	25	570	24	11
Little Caesar's 14" Round Veggie Pizza*	190		7	3	15	500	25	9
Little Caesar's 12" Thin Crust Cheese Pizza*	120		6	2.5	15	280	12	6
Little Caesar's 12" Thin Crust Pepperoni Pizza*	150		8	3.5	20	380	12	7

Item	Calories		Fat	Sat Fat	Chol	Sodium	Carbs	
Little Caesar's 14" Thin Crust Cheese Pizza*	130		6	2.5	15	320	13	6
Little Caesar's 14" Thin Crust Pepperoni Pizza*	160		9	3.5	20	420	13	7
Little Caesar's 16" Round Cheese Pizza*	230		8	3.5	20	440	30	11
Little Caesar's 16" Round Pepperoni Pizza*	260		11	4.5	25	570	31	12
Little Caesar's 18" Round Cheese Pizza*	240		8	3.5	20	470	32	12
Little Caesar's 18" Round Pepperoni Pizza*	270		11	4.5	30	600	32	13
Little Caesar's 12" Deep Dish Cheese Pizza*	140		5	2	10	280	19	7
Little Caesar's 12" Deep Dish Pepperoni Pizza*	160		6	2.5	15	350	19	8
Little Caesar's 14" Deep Dish Cheese Pizza*	140		5	2	10	280	19	7
Little Caesar's 14" Deep Dish Pepperoni Pizza*	160		7	2.5	15	350	19	8
Little Caesar's Cheese Pizza By The Slice	290		10	4.5	25	570	39	14
Little Caesar's Pepperoni Pizza By The Slice	340		14	6	35	770	39	16
Little Caesar's Crazy Bread (1 slice)	90		2.5	0.5	0	120	14	3
Little Caesar's Crazy Sauce	45		0	0	0	250	9	1
Little Caesar's Baby Pan! Pan!	310		15	5.5	30	640	32	14
Little Caesar's Italian Cheese Bread (1 piece)	120		6	2	10	240	12	5
Little Caesar's Chicken Wings (1 wing)	50		4	1	15	640	0	4
Little Caesar's Cinnamon Caesar Stick	340		9	1	0	440	57	8
Little Caesar's Deli Italian Sandwich	690		32	13	75	1730	68	34
Little Caesar's Deli Veggie Sandwich	720		38	11.5	30	1240	71	26
Little Caesar's Deli Ham and Cheese Sandwich	600		22	9.5	55	1480	68	33
Little Caesar's Tossed Side Salad	50		0.5	0	0	60	9	2

123

Little Caesar's Antipasto Salad	130		7	3.5	15	390	10	7
Little Caesar's Italian Dressing	210		22	3	0	360	2	0
Little Caesar's Ranch Dressing	270		29	5	4	380	1	0
Little Caesar's Fat Free Italian Dressing	25		0	0	0	390	5	0

* Single Slice

Long John Silver's Menu	Total Calories	Fat Calories	Total Fat (g)	Sat. Fat (g)	Chol. (mg)	Sodium (mg)	Carbs (g)	Protein (g)
Long John Silver's Ultimate Fish Sandwich	480	220	25	10	50	1400	46	19
Long John Silver's Fish Sandwich	430	180	20	5	35	1150	46	16
Long John Silver's Fish Sandwich w/ Cheese	480	220	25	10	50	1390	46	16
Long John Silver's Regular Battered Fish	230	120	13	4	30	700	16	12
Long John Silver's Country Style Breaded Fish	200	90	10	1.5	10	300	17	10
Long John Silver's Battered Shrimp	45	25	2.5	1	15	125	3	2
Long John Silver's Breaded Clams	250	130	14	3.5	35	560	26	9
Long John Silver's Lemon Crumb Fish (2)	240	110	12	4	55	1490	52	27
Long John Silver's Popcorn Shrimp	320	130	15	2.5	85	1440	33	15
Long John Silver's Crabcake	150	80	9	2	15	180	12	4
Long John Silver's Chicken Sandwich	340	130	14	3.5	25	840	40	13
Long John Silver's Chicken Sandwich w/ Cheese	390	170	19	9	40	1090	40	16
Long John Silver's Battered Chicken Plank	140	70	8	2.5	20	400	9	8
Long John Silver's Ocean Chef Salad	130	20	2	0	60	540	15	14
Long John Silver's Grilled Chicken Salad	140	20	2.5	0.5	45	260	10	20
Long John Silver's Garden Salad	45	0	0	0	0	25	9	3

Long John Silver's Side Salad	20	0	0	0	0	10	3	1
Long John Silver's Broccoli Cheese Soup	180	110	12	4.5	15	1240	13	5
Long John Silver's Clam Chowder Cup	260	110	12	5	35	1020	26	12
Long John Silver's Clam Chowder Bowl	520	210	24	10	70	2030	52	24
Long John Silver's French Fries (regular)	250	130	15	2.5	0	500	28	3
Long John Silver's French Fries (large)	420	220	24	4	0	830	46	5
Long John Silver's Hushpuppie	60	20	2.5	0	0	25	9	1
Long John Silver's Cole Slaw (4 ounces)	170	70	7	0	0	310	23	2
Long John Silver's Corn Cobbette	80	5	0.5	0	0	0	19	3
Long John Silver's Corn Cobbette w/ Butter	140	70	8	1.5	0	0	19	3
Long John Silver's Rice	180	40	4	0.5	0	560	34	3
Long John Silver's Cheesesticks	160	80	9	4	10	360	12	6
Long John Silver's Pineapple Creme Cheesecake*	310	150	17	9	5	105	36	4
Long John Silver's Chocolate Creme*	280	150	17	8	15	125	29	4
Long John Silver's Double Lemon*	350	160	18	10	40	180	41	6
Long John Silver's Strawberries N' Creme*	280	130	15	8	15	130	32	4
Long John Silver's Banana Split Sundae*	300	150	17	9	15	130	34	4
Long John Silver's Pecan*	390	170	19	4	40	250	53	3
Long John Silver's Dutch Apple*	290	110	13	4	0	250	44	2
Long John Silver's Coke (medium)	270	0	0	0	0	20	62	0
Long John Silver's Diet Coke (medium)	0	0	0	0	0	25	0	0
Long John Silver's Dr. Pepper (medium)	250	0	0	0	0	60	69	0
Long John Silver's Sprite (med)	260	0	0	0	0	55	62	0

	Total Calories	Fat Calories	Total Fat (g)	Sat. Fat (g)	Chol. (mg)	Sodium (mg)	Carbs (g)	Protein (g)
Long John Silver's Hi-C Pink Lemonade (medium)	260	0	0	0	0	110	62	0
Long John Silver's Minute Maid Lemonade (medium)	260	0	0	0	0	110	69	0

* a suggested serving size of 1 slice

McDonalds Menu	Total Calories	Fat Calories	Total Fat (g)	Sat. Fat (g)	Chol. (mg)	Sodium (mg)	Carbs (g)	Protein (g)
McDonald's Biscuit	240	100	11	2.5	0	640	30	4
McDonald's Breakfast Burrito	290	150	16	6	170	680	24	13
McDonald's Apple Danish	340	130	15	3	20	340	47	5
McDonald's Cheese Danish	400	190	21	5	40	400	45	7
McDonald's Cinnamon Roll	390	160	18	5	65	310	50	6
McDonald's Scrambled Eggs (2)	160	100	11	3.5	425	170	1	13
McDonald's English Muffin	140	20	2	0	0	210	25	4
McDonald's Hash Browns	130	70	8	1.5	0	330	14	1
McDonald's Lowfat Apple Bran Muffin	300	30	3	0.5	0	380	61	6
McDonald's Hotcakes (plain)	340	70	8	1.5	20	630	58	9
McDonald's Hotcakes (margarine 2 pats & syrup)	600	150	17	3	20	770	104	9
McDonald's Egg McMuffin	290	110	12	4.5	235	790	27	17
McDonald's Sausage McMuffin	360	210	23	8	45	740	26	13
McDonald's Sausage McMuffin w/ Egg	440	250	28	10	255	890	27	19
McDonald's Sausage Biscuit	410	250	28	8	35	930	30	10
McDonald's Sausage Biscuit w/ Egg	490	300	33	10	245	1010	31	16
McDonald's Bacon, Egg & Cheese Biscuit	480	280	31	10	250	1410	31	20
McDonald's Ham & Egg Cheese Bagel	550	210	23	8	255	1490	58	26
McDonald's Spanish Omelet Bagel	690	350	38	14	275	1570	60	27
McDonald's Steak & Egg Cheese Bagel	700	320	35	13	290	1290	57	38
McDonald's Sausage	170	150	16	5	35	290	0	6

McDonald's Cheeseburger	330	130	14	6	45	830	36	15
McDonald's Quarter Pounder	430	190	21	8	70	840	37	23
McDonald's Quarter Pounder w/ Cheese	530	270	30	13	95	1310	38	28
McDonald's Big Mac	590	310	34	11	85	1090	47	24
McDonald's Big N' Tasty	540	290	32	10	80	970	39	24
McDonald's Big N' Tasty w/ Cheese	590	330	37	12	95	1210	40	27
McDonald's Crispy Chicken	550	240	27	4.5	50	1180	54	23
McDonald's Chicken McGrill	450	160	18	3	60	970	46	26
McDonald's Chicken McNuggets (4)	190	100	11	2.5	35	360	13	10
McDonald's Chicken McNuggets (6)	290	150	17	3.5	55	540	20	15
McDonald's Chicken McNuggets (9)	430	220	25	5	80	810	29	23
McDonald's Filet-O-Fish	470	240	26	5	50	1200	67	24
McDonald's Chef Salad	150	70	8	3.5	95	740	5	17
McDonald's Garden Salad	100	60	6	3	75	120	4	7
McDonald's Grilled Chicken Caesar Salad	100	25	2.5	1.5	40	240	3	17
McDonald's French Fries (small)	210	90	10	1.5	0	135	26	3
McDonald's French Fries (medium)	450	200	22	4	0	290	57	6
McDonald's French Fries (large)	540	230	26	4.5	0	350	68	8
McDonald's French Fries (super size)	610	260	29	5	0	390	77	9
McDonald's Chocolate Chip Cookie	280	130	14	8	40	170	37	3
McDonald's McDonaldland Cookies	230	70	8	2	0	250	38	3
McDonald's Vanilla Reduced Fat Ice Cream Cone	150	40	4.5	3	20	75	23	4
McDonald's Strawberry Sundae	290	70	7	5	30	95	50	7
McDonald's Hot Caramel Sundae	360	90	10	6	35	180	61	7
McDonald's Hot Fudge Sundae	340	100	12	9	30	170	52	8
McDonald's Nuts (Sundaes)	40	30	3.5	0	0	55	2	2

	Total Calories	Fat Calories	Total Fat (g)	Sat. Fat (g)	Chol. (mg)	Sodium (mg)	Carbs (g)	Protein (g)
McDonald's Butterfinger® McFlurry	620	190	22	14	70	260	90	16
McDonald's M&M® McFlurry	630	200	23	15	75	210	90	16
McDonald's Nestle Crunch® McFlurry	630	220	24	16	75	230	89	16
McDonald's Oreo® McFlurry	570	180	20	12	70	280	82	15
McDonald's Baked Apple Pie	260	120	13	3.5	0	200	34	3
McDonald's Fruit 'n Yogurt Parfait	380	50	5	2	15	240	76	10
McDonald's Fruit 'n Yogurt Parfait (no granola)	280	35	4	2	15	115	53	8
McDonald's Vanilla Shake (small)	360	80	9	6	40	250	59	11
McDonald's Chocolate Shake (small)	360	80	9	6	40	250	60	11
McDonald's Strawberry Shake (small)	360	80	9	6	40	180	60	11
McDonald's Coca Cola Classic (small)	150	0	0	0	0	15	40	0
McDonald's Diet Coke (small)	0	0	0	0	0	20	0	0
McDonald's Sprite (small)	150	0	0	0	0	55	39	0
McDonald's Hi-C Orange Drink (small)	160	0	0	0	0	30	44	0
McDonald's Orange Juice	80	0	0	0	0	20	20	0
McDonald's Milk (1% fat)	100	20	2.5	1.5	10	115	13	8

Pizza Hut Menu	Total Calories	Fat Calories	Total Fat (g)	Sat. Fat (g)	Chol. (mg)	Sodium (mg)	Carbs (g)	Protein (g)
Pizza Hut Big New Yorker Cheese	380	150	17	9	20	1140	41	19
Pizza Hut Big New Yorker Pepperoni	370	150	16	7	20	1150	41	17
Pizza Hut Big New Yorker Ham	340	120	13	6	25	1160	41	18
Pizza Hut Big New Yorker Beef Topping	480	230	26	11	40	1380	42	24
Pizza Hut Big New Yorker Pork Topping	470	220	25	10	35	1470	42	23
Pizza Hut Big New Yorker Sausage	570	300	33	14	55	1620	42	27

Pizza Hut Big New Yorker Supreme	450	200	23	10	35	1350	43	22
Pizza Hut Big New Yorker Veggie Lover's Pizza	450	200	22	6	10	1340	52	18
Pizza Hut The Edge The Works	110	50	6	2.5	10	270	9	5
Pizza Hut The Edge Veggie Lover's	70	25	3	1.5	<5	180	9	4
Pizza Hut The Edge Meat Lover's	160	100	11	4.5	20	440	8	7
Pizza Hut The Edge Chicken Supreme	90	30	3.5	1.5	15	290	9	7
Pizza Hut Pan Pizza Cheese	290	130	14	6	10	590	28	12
Pizza Hut Pan Pizza Beef Topping	330	160	18	7	20	690	29	14
Pizza Hut Pan Pizza Ham	260	100	12	4	15	610	28	11
Pizza Hut Pan Pizza Pepperoni	280	130	14	5	15	610	28	11
Pizza Hut Pan Pizza Italian Sausage	340	180	20	7	25	720	29	13
Pizza Hut Pan Pizza Pork Topping	320	160	17	6	20	730	29	13
Pizza Hut Pan Pizza Meat Lover's	360	190	21	7	30	840	29	14
Pizza Hut Pan Pizza Veggie Lover's	270	110	12	4	5	510	30	10
Pizza Hut Pan Pizza Pepperoni Lover's	330	160	18	7	20	760	29	14
Pizza Hut Pan Pizza Supreme	320	150	17	6	20	670	29	13
Pizza Hut Pan Pizza Super Supreme	340	170	18	6	25	780	30	14
Pizza Hut Pan Pizza Chicken Supreme	270	100	12	4	15	580	29	13
Pizza Hut Hand Tossed Pizza Cheese	240	90	10	5	10	650	28	12
Pizza Hut Hand Tossed Pizza Beef Topping	330	150	17	8	25	880	29	16
Pizza Hut Hand Tossed Pizza Ham	260	90	10	5	20	800	28	14
Pizza Hut Hand Tossed Pizza Pepperoni	280	110	13	6	20	790	28	13
Pizza Hut Hand Tossed Pizza Italian Sausage	340	170	18	8	30	910	28	16

Pizza Hut Hand Tossed Pizza Pork Topping	320	150	16	7	25	920	29	16
Pizza Hut Hand Tossed Pizza Meat Lover's	320	150	17	7	30	900	28	14
Pizza Hut Hand Tossed Pizza Veggie Lover's	220	70	8	3	5	580	29	9
Pizza Hut Hand Tossed Pizza Pepperoni Lover's	250	100	11	4.5	15	730	27	11
Pizza Hut Hand Tossed Pizza Supreme	270	110	12	5	20	730	29	13
Pizza Hut Hand Tossed Pizza Super Supreme	290	130	14	6	25	850	29	13
Pizza Hut Hand Tossed Pizza Chicken Supreme	230	60	7	3.5	15	650	29	13
Pizza Hut Sicilian Cheese	290	120	13	6	10	630	31	12
Pizza Hut Sicilian Beef Topping	260	100	11	4.5	15	640	31	11
Pizza Hut Sicilian Ham	257	92	10	4.9	14	745	30	11
Pizza Hut Sicilian Pepperoni	280	120	13	5	15	630	31	10
Pizza Hut Sicilian Italian Sausage	333	158	18	7.4	24	855	31	13
Pizza Hut Sicilian Pork Topping	320	140	16	6	20	750	31	13
Pizza Hut Sicilian Meat Lover's	350	170	19	7	25	830	31	14
Pizza Hut Sicilian Veggies Lover's	270	100	11	4	15	620	32	12
Pizza Hut Sicilian Pepperoni Lover's	320	150	16	7	20	780	31	13
Pizza Hut Sicilian Supreme	310	140	15	6	15	690	32	12
Pizza Hut Sicilian Super Supreme	340	160	18	6	20	780	32	13
Pizza Hut Sicilian Chicken Supreme	270	100	11	4	15	620	32	12
Pizza Hut Stuffed Crust Cheese	445	174	19	9.9	24	1090	46	22
Pizza Hut Stuffed Crust Beef Topping	466	193	22	10.2	30	1137	46	23
Pizza Hut Stuffed Crust Ham	404	199	22	12.3	39	1190	45	24
Pizza Hut Stuffed Crust Pepperoni	438	173	19	9.1	27	1116	45	21
Pizza Hut Stuffed Crust Italian Sausage	478	206	23	10.3	35	1164	46	22

Pizza Hut Stuffed Crust Pork Topping	461	192	21	9.7	29	1176	46	22
Pizza Hut Stuffed Crust Meat Lover's	543	256	29	12.5	48	1427	46	26
Pizza Hut Stuffed Crust Veggie Lover's	421	145	17	8	19	1039	48	20
Pizza Hut Stuffed Crust Pepperoni Lover's	525	236	26	12.5	40	1413	46	26
Pizza Hut Stuffed Crust Supreme	487	207	23	10.5	33	1227	47	24
Pizza Hut Stuffed Crust Super Supreme	505	226	25	11	44	1371	46	25
Pizza Hut Stuffed Crust Chicken Supreme	432	148	17	8.1	32	1111	47	24
Pizza Hut Thin 'n Crispy Cheese	200	80	9	5	10	590	22	10
Pizza Hut Thin 'n Crispy Beef Topping	270	130	15	7	25	750	22	13
Pizza Hut Thin 'n Crispy Ham	170	60	7	3.5	15	610	21	9
Pizza Hut Thin 'n Crispy Pepperoni	190	80	9	4	15	610	21	9
Pizza Hut Thin 'n Crispy Italian Sausage	290	150	17	7	30	800	22	12
Pizza Hut Thin 'n Crispy Pork Topping	270	130	14	6	25	820	22	13
Pizza Hut Thin 'n Crispy Meat Lover's	310	170	19	8	35	910	22	14
Pizza Hut Thin 'n Crispy Veggie Lover's	190	70	7	3	5	520	24	8
Pizza Hut Thin 'n Crispy Pepperoni Lover's	250	110	13	6	20	760	22	12
Pizza Hut Thin 'n Crispy Supreme	250	120	13	6	20	710	23	12
Pizza Hut Thin 'n Crispy Super Supreme	280	140	15	6	25	840	23	13
Pizza Hut Thin 'n Crispy Chicken Supreme	200	60	7	3.5	20	620	23	12
Pizza Hut Personal Pan Pizza Cheese	630	250	28	12	25	1370	71	28
Pizza Hut Personal Pan Pizza Pepperoni	620	250	28	11	30	1430	70	26

	Total Calories	Fat Calories	Total Fat (g)	Saturated Fat (g)	Cholest (mg)	Sodium (mg)	Carbs (g)	Protein (g)
Pizza Hut Personal Pan Pizza Ham	580	210	23	9	35	1450	70	27
Pizza Hut Personal Pan Pizza Beef Topping	710	320	35	14	45	1580	71	31
Pizza Hut Personal Pan Pizza Pork Topping	700	310	34	13	40	1670	71	31
Pizza Hut Personal Pan Pizza Italian Sausage	740	350	39	14	55	1640	71	31
Pizza Hut Spaghetti w/ Marinara	490	50	6	1	0	730	91	18
Pizza Hut Spaghetti w/ Meat Sauce	600	120	13	5	8	910	98	23
Pizza Hut Spaghette w/ Meatballs	850	220	24	10	17	1120	120	37
Pizza Hut Cavatini Pasta	480	130	14	6	8	1170	66	21
Pizza Hut Cavatini Supreme Pasta	560	170	19	8	10	1400	73	24
Pizza Hut Ham & Cheese Sandwich	550	190	21	7	22	2150	57	33
Pizza Hut Supreme Sandwich	640	250	28	10	28	2150	62	34
Pizza Hut Mild Buffalo Wings (5)	200	110	12	3.5	150	510	<1	23
Pizza Hut Hot Buffalo Wings (4)	210	110	12	3	130	900	4	22
Pizza Hut Garlic Bread (1 Slice)	150	70	8	1.5	0	240	16	3
Pizza Hut Bread Stick (1 Serving)	130	35	4	1	0	170	20	3
Pizza Hut Bread Stick Dipping Sauce (1 Serving)	30	5	0.5	0	0	170	5	<1
Pizza Hut Apple Dessert Pizza (1 Slice)	250	40	4.5	1	0	230	48	3
Pizza Hut Cherry Dessert Pizza (1 Slice)	250	40	4.5	1	0	220	47	3

Sonic Drive-In Menu	Total Calories	Fat Calories	Total Fat (g)	Saturated Fat (g)	Cholest (mg)	Sodium (mg)	Carbs (g)	Protein (g)
Sonic Drive-In No. 1 Burger	577	325	36	7	37	753	43	14
Sonic Drive-In No. 2 Burger	481	225	25	5	29	761	43	14
Sonic Drive-In No. 1 Cheeseburger	647	379	42	11	52	1103	44	18

	Total Calories	Fat Calories	Total Fat (g)	Sat. Fat (g)	Chol. (mg)	Sodium (mg)	Carbs (g)	Protein (g)
Sonic Drive-In No. 2 Cheeseburger	551	279	31	9	44	1111	44	18
Sonic Drive-In Bacon Cheeseburger	727	442	49	13	67	1433	44	23
Sonic Drive-In Super Sonic No. 1	929	596	66	19	96	1476	45	28
Sonic Drive-In Super Sonic No. 2	839	496	55	17	88	1571	46	28
Sonic Drive-In Jr. Burger	353	192	21	6	45	1294	27	14

Subway Menu	Total Calories	Fat Calories	Total Fat (g)	Sat. Fat (g)	Chol. (mg)	Sodium (mg)	Carbs (g)	Protein (g)
Subway Classic 6" BMT	453	216	24	8	56	1740	40	21
Subway Classic 6" Cold Cut Trio	415	184	20	7	57	1670	40	19
Subway Classic 6" Meatball	501	228	25	10	56	1350	46	23
Subway Classic 6" Seafood & Crab	378	141	16	4.5	24	1270	46	14
Subway Classic 6" Steak & Cheese	362	117	13	4.5	37	1200	41	23
Subway Classic 6" Subway Melt	384	136	15	5	44	1720	40	22
Subway Classic 6" Tuna	419	190	21	5	42	1180	39	18
Subway Select 6" Asiago Caesar Chicken	391	138	15	3	47	1000	41	22
Subway Select 6" Caesar Italian BMT	530	285	31	10	66	1840	41	22
Subway Select 6" Honey Mustard Melt	376	103	11	5	44	1590	47	22
Subway Select 6" Honey Mustard Turkey w/ Cucumber	275	32	3.5	1	20	990	46	16
Subway Select 6" Horseradish Roast Beef	401	154	17	3	27	880	42	18
Subway Select 6" Horseradish Steak & Cheese	468	198	22	6	44	1110	43	22
Subway Select 6" Southwest Chicken	362	118	13	2.5	43	960	40	21
Subway Select 6" Southwest Steak & Cheese	412	165	18	6	44	1120	42	22
Subway 6" Ham	261	40	4.5	1.5	25	1260	39	17

	Total Calories	Fat Calories	Total Fat (g)	Sat. Fat (g)	Chol. (mg)	Sodium (mg)	Carbs (g)	Protein (g)
Subway 6" Roast Beef	264	41	4.5	1	20	840	39	18
Subway 6" Roasted Chicken Breast	311	51	6	1.5	48	880	40	25
Subway 6" Subway Club	294	46	5	1.5	33	1250	40	22
Subway 6" Turkey Breast	254	34	3.5	1	20	1000	39	16
Subway 6" Turkey Breast & Ham	267	39	4.5	1	26	1210	40	18
Subway 6" Veggie Delite	200	23	2.5	0.5	0	500	37	7
Subway Deli Ham Sandwich	194	32	3.5	1	12	750	30	10
Subway Deli Roast Beef Sandwich	206	36	4	1	13	600	31	12
Subway Deli Tuna Sandwich	309	138	15	4	26	810	31	12
Subway Deli Turkey Breast Sandwich	200	31	3.5	1	13	700	31	12
Subway Asiago Caesar Chicken Wrap	413	137	15	3	47	1320	47	22
Subway Steak and Cheese Wrap	353	84	9	4	37	1400	46	22
Subway Turkey Breast & Bacon Wrap	321	67	7	2.5	28	1510	45	18

Taco Bell Menu	Total Calories	Fat Calories	Total Fat (g)	Sat. Fat (g)	Chol. (mg)	Sodium (mg)	Carbs (g)	Protein (g)
Taco Bell Taco	210	110	12	4	30	330	18	9
Taco Bell Taco Supreme	260	140	16	6	40	350	20	10
Taco Bell Soft Taco - Beef	210	90	10	4	30	570	20	11
Taco Bell Soft Taco - Chicken	190	60	7	2.5	35	480	19	13
Taco Bell Soft Taco - Steak	280	150	17	4	35	630	20	12
Taco Bell Double Decker Taco	380	150	17	5	30	740	43	15
Taco Bell Double Decker Taco Supreme	420	180	21	8	40	760	45	15
Taco Bell Bean Burrito	370	110	12	3.5	10	1080	54	13
Taco Bell 7-Layer Burrito	520	200	22	7	25	1270	65	16
Taco Bell Chili Cheese Burrito	330	120	13	5	25	900	40	13
Taco Bell Burrito Supreme - Beef	430	170	18	7	40	1210	50	17
Taco Bell Burrito Supreme - Chicken	410	140	16	6	45	1120	49	20

Taco Bell Burrito Supreme - Steak	420	140	16	6	35	1140	48	21
Taco Bell Double Burrito Supreme - Beef	510	210	23	9	60	1500	52	23
Taco Bell Double Burrito Supreme - Chicken	460	150	17	6	70	1200	50	27
Taco Bell Double Burrito Supreme - Steak	470	160	18	7	55	1230	48	28
Taco Bell Fiesta Burrito - Beef	380	130	15	5	30	1100	49	14
Taco Bell Fiesta Burrito - Chicken	370	110	12	3.5	35	1000	48	17
Taco Bell Fiesta Burrito - Steak	370	110	12	4	25	1020	47	18
Taco Bell Grilled Stuft Burrito - Beef	730	320	35	11	65	2090	75	27
Taco Bell Grilled Stuft Burrito - Chicken	690	270	29	8	70	1900	73	33
Taco Bell Grilled Stuft Burrito - Steak	690	270	30	8	60	1970	72	30
Taco Bell Chalupa Supreme - Beef	380	200	23	8	40	580	29	14
Taco Bell Chalupa Supreme - Chicken	360	180	20	7	45	490	28	17
Taco Bell Chalupa Supreme - Steak	360	180	20	7	35	500	27	17
Taco Bell Chalupa Baja - Beef	420	240	27	7	35	760	30	14
Taco Bell Chalupa Baja - Chicken	400	210	24	5	40	660	28	17
Taco Bell Chalupa Baja - Steak	400	220	24	6	30	680	27	17
Taco Bell Chalupa Nacho Cheese - Beef	370	200	22	6	25	740	30	13
Taco Bell Chalupa Nacho Cheese - Chicken	350	170	19	4.5	25	640	29	16
Taco Bell Chalupa Nacho Cheese - Steak	350	170	19	4.5	20	660	28	16
Taco Bell Chalupa Santa Fe - Beef	440	260	29	7	35	660	31	14
Taco Bell Chalupa Santa Fe - Chicken	420	240	26	6	40	560	30	17
Taco Bell Chalupa Santa Fe - Steak	430	240	27	6	35	580	29	18

Taco Bell Gordita Supreme - Beef	300	120	14	5	35	550	27	17
Taco Bell Gordita Supreme - Chicken	300	120	13	5	45	530	28	16
Taco Bell Gordita Supreme - Steak	300	120	14	5	35	550	27	17
Taco Bell Gordita Baja - Beef	360	190	21	5	35	810	29	13
Taco Bell Gordita Baja - Chicken	340	160	18	4	40	710	28	16
Taco Bell Gordita Baja - Steak	340	160	18	4	35	760	28	15
Taco Bell Gordita Nacho Cheese - Beef	310	140	15	4	25	780	30	13
Taco Bell Gordita Nacho Cheese - Chicken	290	110	13	2.5	25	690	29	15
Taco Bell Gordita Nacho Cheese - Steak	290	120	13	3	20	700	28	16
Taco Bell Gordita Santa Fe - Beef	380	210	23	5	35	700	31	14
Taco Bell Gordita Santa Fe - Chicken	370	180	20	4	40	610	30	17
Taco Bell Gordita Santa Fe - Steak	370	180	20	4.5	35	620	29	17
Taco Bell Cheesy Gordita Crunch	560	300	33	11	60	980	44	21
Taco Bell Cheesy Gordita Crunch Supreme	610	340	37	13	70	990	47	22
Taco Bell Nachos	320	160	18	4	<5	560	34	5
Taco Bell Nachos Supreme	440	210	24	7	35	800	44	14
Taco Bell Nachos BellGrande	760	350	39	11	35	1300	83	20
Taco Bell Mucho Grande Nachos	1320	740	82	25	75	2670	116	31
Taco Bell Pintos'n Cheese	180	80	8	4	15	640	18	9
Taco Bell Mexican Rice	190	80	9	3.5	15	750	23	5
Taco Bell Cinnamon Twists	150	40	4.5	1	0	190	27	1
Taco Bell Tostada	250	110	12	4.5	15	640	27	10
Taco Bell Mexican Pizza	390	220	25	8	45	930	28	18
Taco Bell Enchirito - Beef	370	170	19	9	50	1300	33	18
Taco Bell Enchirito - Chicken	350	140	16	8	55	1210	32	21
Taco Bell Enchirito - Steak	350	150	16	8	45	1220	31	22

	Total Calories	Fat Calories	Total Fat (g)	Sat. Fat (g)	Chol. (mg)	Sodium (mg)	Carbs (g)	Protein (g)
Taco Bell MexiMelt	290	140	15	7	45	830	22	15
Taco Bell Taco Salad with Salsa	850	470	52	14	70	2250	69	30
Taco Bell Taco Salad with Salsa without Shell	400	200	22	10	70	1510	31	24
Taco Bell Cheese Quesadilla	350	160	18	9	50	860	31	16
Taco Bell Chicken Quesadilla	400	180	19	9	75	1050	33	25

Wendy's Menu	Total Calories	Fat Calories	Total Fat (g)	Sat. Fat (g)	Chol. (mg)	Sodium (mg)	Carbs (g)	Protein (g)
Wendy's Classic Single w/ Everything	410	170	19	7	70	920	37	25
Wendy's Big Bacon Classic	580	270	30	12	100	1460	46	34
Wendy's Jr. Hamburger	270	80	9	3	30	620	34	14
Wendy's Jr. Cheeseburger	310	110	12	6	45	800	34	17
Wendy's Jr. Bacon Cheeseburger	380	170	19	7	55	870	34	20
Wendy's Jr. Cheeseburger Deluxe	350	140	16	6	50	860	36	18
Wendy's Grilled Chicken Sandwich	300	60	7	1.5	55	740	36	24
Wendy's Chicken Breast Fillet Sandwich	430	150	16	3	55	750	46	27
Wendy's Chicken Club Sandwich	470	180	20	4.5	65	940	47	30
Wendy's Spicy Chicken Sandwich	410	120	14	2.5	65	1280	43	28
Wendy's Crispy Chicken Nuggets (5)	230	140	16	3	30	470	11	11
Wendy's Crispy Chicken Nuggets (4)	190	120	13	2.5	25	380	9	9
Wendy's Barbecue Sauce	45	0	0	0	0	160	10	1
Wendy's Honey Mustard Sauce	130	100	12	2	10	220	6	0
Wendy's Sweet and Sour Sauce	50	0	0	0	0	120	12	0
Wendy's Caesar Side Salad	110	50	5	2.5	15	380	6	9
Wendy's Side Salad	60	25	3	0.5	0	160	5	4
Wendy's Deluxe Garden Salad	110	50	6	1	0	320	10	7
Wendy's Grilled Chicken Salad	200	60	7	1.5	55	780	10	27

Wendy's Taco Salad	380	170	19	10	65	1040	28	26
Wendy's Taco Chips	210	80	9	1.5	0	160	28	3
Wendy's Soft Breadstick	130	30	3	0.5	5	250	23	4
Wendy's Blue Cheese Dressing	360	350	38	7	30	350	1	2
Wendy's French Dressing	250	190	21	3	0	670	13	0
Wendy's French Dressing, Fat Free	70	0	0	0	0	300	18	0
Wendy's Italian Caesar Dressing	230	220	24	4	25	350	1	1
Wendy's Italian Dressing, Reduced Fat	80	60	7	1	0	690	6	0
Wendy's Hidden Valley Ranch Dressing	200	180	20	3	25	410	3	1
Wendy's Hidden Valley Ranch Dressing, Reduced Fat	120	100	11	2	20	470	4	1
Wendy's Thousand Island Dressing	260	230	25	4	20	380	7	1
Wendy's French Fries (kids)	270	120	13	2	0	85	35	4
Wendy's French Fries (medium)	420	180	20	3	0	130	55	6
Wendy's French Fries (biggie)	470	200	23	3.5	0	150	61	7
Wendy's French Fries (great biggie)	570	240	27	4	0	180	73	8
Wendy's Plain Baked Potato	310	0	0	0	0	25	72	7
Wendy's Bacon & Cheese Baked Potato	530	160	17	4	25	820	78	16
Wendy's Broccoli & Cheese Baked Potato	470	130	14	3	5	470	80	9
Wendy's Sour Cream & Chive Baked Potato	370	50	5	4	15	75	72	7
Wendy's Whipped Margarine	70	60	7	1.5	0	115	0	0
Wendy's Chili (small)	210	60	7	2.5	30	800	21	15
Wendy's Chili (large)	310	90	10	3.5	45	1190	32	23
Wendy's Shredded Cheddar Cheese	70	50	6	3.5	15	110	1	4
Wendy's Saltine Crackers	25	5	0.5	0	0	80	4	1
Wendy's Frosty (junior)	170	40	4	2.5	20	100	26	4
Wendy's Frosty (small)	330	80	8	5	35	200	56	8
Wendy's Frosty (medium)	440	100	11	7	50	260	73	11

	Total Calories	Fat Calories	Total Fat (g)	Saturated Fat (g)	Cholest (mg)	Sodium (mg)	Carbs (g)	Protein (g)
Wendy's Cola Soft Drink	130	0	0	0	0	10	36	0
Wendy's Diet Cola Soft Drink	0	0	0	0	0	15	0	0
Wendy's Lemon-Lime Soft Drink	130	0	0	0	0	30	34	0

White Castle Menu	Total Calories	Fat Calories	Total Fat (g)	Saturated Fat (g)	Cholest (mg)	Sodium (mg)	Carbs (g)	Protein (g)
White Castle Hamburger	135	65	7	3	10	135	11	6
White Castle Cheeseburger	160	85	9	4	15	250	11	7
White Castle Double Hamburger	235	125	14	6	20	200	16	11
White Castle Double Cheeseburger	285	165	18	8	30	430	16	14
White Castle Bacon Cheeseburger	200	115	13	6	25	400	12	10
White Castle Fish Sandwich	160	60	6	1	15	220	18	8
White Castle Chicken Ring Sandwich	170	70	7	1	24	210	5	5
White Castle Breakfast Sandwich	340	220	25	10	130	900	17	14
White Castle Chicken Rings (6)	310	190	21	4	70	620	14	16
White Castle Onion Rings (8)	460		27			550	56	12
White Castle French Fries (small)	115	50	6	1	0	15	15	
White Castle Cheese Sticks	491	249	28	8	0	1216	32	25
White Castle Coca-Cola Classic (20 ounces)	171	0	0	0	0	17	46	0
White Castle Diet Coke (20 ounces)	1	0	0	0	0	19	0	0
White Castle Coffee (12 ounces)	6	0	0	0	0	5	1	0
White Castle Iced Tea (14 ounces)	45	0	0	0	0	15	12	0

	Total Calories	Fat Calories	Total Fat (g)	Sat. Fat (g)	Chol. (mg)	Sodium (mg)	Carbs (g)	Protein (g)
White Castle Vanilla Shake (14 ounces)	230	60	7	1	25	150	35	8
White Castle Chocolate Shake (14 ounces)	220	60	7	1	25	140	32	8

Wienerschnitzel Menu	Total Calories	Fat Calories	Total Fat (g)	Sat. Fat (g)	Chol. (mg)	Sodium (mg)	Carbs (g)	Protein (g)
Wienerschnitzel Original Mustard Dog	258	124	14	5	21	794		
Wienerschnitzel Original Chili Dog	295	148	16	5	28	935		
Wienerschnitzel Original Chili Cheese Dog	348	188	21	8	41	1137		
Wienerschnitzel Original Kraut Dog	265	122	14	5	21	1148		
Wienerschnitzel Original Deluxe Dog	275	124	14	5	21	1621		
Wienerschnitzel Original Relish Dog	279	124	14	5	21	902		
Wienerschnitzel Original BBQ Bacon Dog	378	208	23	9	43	985		
Wienerschnitzel Corn Dog	290	203	23	8	26	460		
Wienerschnitzel Fries (regular)	270	189	21	13	30	461		
Wienerschnitzel French Fries (large)	379	265	29	17	42	690		
Wienerschnitzel Chili Cheese Fries	466	326	36	19	64	1001		
Wienerschnitzel Deluxe Hamburger	576	334	37	12	90	1145		
Wienerschnitzel Deluxe Cheeseburger	635	375	42	14	103	1350		
Wienerschnitzel Deluxe Bacon Cheeseburger	686	412	46	16	110	1519		
Wienerschnitzel Chicken Deluxe	536	289	32	9	48	961		
Wienerschnitzel Breakfast Burrito	571	331	37	13	526	1103		
Wienerschnitzel Breakfast Sandwich	446	250	27	10	285	1040		

Web Guide

Online BMI Calculator: http://www.nhlbisupport.com/bmi/

Further Reading

Sly Moves – Sylvester Stallone
Eat This, Not That – David Zinczenko/Matt Goulding
Eat This Not That! Supermarket Survival Guide: The No-Diet
    Weight Loss Solution - David Zinczenko/Matt Goulding
Cook This, Not That! The Kitchen Survival Guide - David
    Zinczenko/Matt Goulding

Meditation CD's

*Music For Relaxation and Meditation – by MindWaves
    Highly Recommended – uses Brain Wave Synchronization
Deeper Journeys – Steven Halpern
Rasa Live – Rasa
Slow Music For Yoga – Al Gromer Khan

Website Resources:

www.nih.gov – National Institute for Health
www.mypyramid.gov/mypyramid/index.aspx – U.S. Dept. of
    Agriculture Meal Plan Calculator
www.fitness.gov – The President's Council on Physical Fitness
    and Sports
www.ncppa.org – National Coalition for Promoting Physical
    Activity
www.acefitness.org – American Council on Exercise
www.arthritis.org   The Arthritis Foundation offers tips on
    exercising with arthritis
www.justmove.org – Just Move (American Heart Association)
www.nhlbi.nih.gov/health/public/heart/obesity/wecan –
    National Heart, Lung, and Blood Institute)

www.ingramcontent.com/pod-product-compliance
Lightning Source LLC
Chambersburg PA
CBHW052208270326
41931CB00011B/2264